Incorporating Occupational Information in Electronic Health Records

LETTER REPORT

Committee on Occupational Information
and Electronic Health Records

Board on Health Sciences Policy

David H. Wegman, Catharyn T. Liverman,
Andrea M. Schultz, and Larisa M. Strawbridge, *Editors*

INSTITUTE OF MEDICINE
OF THE NATIONAL ACADEMIES

THE NATIONAL ACADEMIES PRESS
Washington, D.C.
www.nap.edu

THE NATIONAL ACADEMIES PRESS • 500 Fifth Street, N.W. • Washington, DC 20001

NOTICE: The project that is the subject of this report was approved by the Governing Board of the National Research Council, whose members are drawn from the councils of the National Academy of Sciences, the National Academy of Engineering, and the Institute of Medicine. The members of the committee responsible for the report were chosen for their special competences and with regard for appropriate balance.

This study was requested by the National Institute for Occupational Safety and Health of the Centers for Disease Control and Prevention and supported by Award No. 211-2006-19152, T.O. #1, between the National Academy of Sciences and the Centers for Disease Control and Prevention. Any opinions, findings, conclusions, or recommendations expressed in this publication are those of the author(s) and do not necessarily reflect the view of the organizations or agencies that provided support for this project.

International Standard Book Number-13: 978-0-309-21743-9
International Standard Book Number-10: 0-309-21743-1

Additional copies of this report are available from the National Academies Press, 500 Fifth Street, N.W., Lockbox 285, Washington, DC 20055; (800) 624-6242 or (202) 334-3313 (in the Washington metropolitan area); Internet, http://www.nap.edu.

For more information about the Institute of Medicine, visit the IOM home page at: **www.iom.edu.**

Copyright 2011 by the National Academy of Sciences. All rights reserved.

Printed in the United States of America

The serpent has been a symbol of long life, healing, and knowledge among almost all cultures and religions since the beginning of recorded history. The serpent adopted as a logotype by the Institute of Medicine is a relief carving from ancient Greece, now held by the Staatliche Museen in Berlin.

Suggested citation: IOM (Institute of Medicine). 2011. *Incorporating occupational information in electronic health records: Letter report.* Washington, DC: The National Academies Press.

*"Knowing is not enough; we must apply.
Willing is not enough; we must do."*
—Goethe

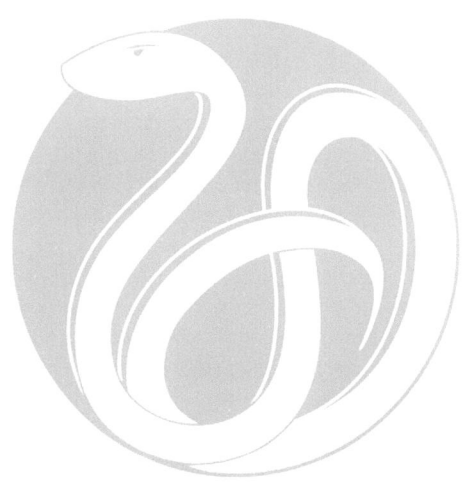

INSTITUTE OF MEDICINE
OF THE NATIONAL ACADEMIES

Advising the Nation. Improving Health.

THE NATIONAL ACADEMIES
Advisers to the Nation on Science, Engineering, and Medicine

The **National Academy of Sciences** is a private, nonprofit, self-perpetuating society of distinguished scholars engaged in scientific and engineering research, dedicated to the furtherance of science and technology and to their use for the general welfare. Upon the authority of the charter granted to it by the Congress in 1863, the Academy has a mandate that requires it to advise the federal government on scientific and technical matters. Dr. Ralph J. Cicerone is president of the National Academy of Sciences.

The **National Academy of Engineering** was established in 1964, under the charter of the National Academy of Sciences, as a parallel organization of outstanding engineers. It is autonomous in its administration and in the selection of its members, sharing with the National Academy of Sciences the responsibility for advising the federal government. The National Academy of Engineering also sponsors engineering programs aimed at meeting national needs, encourages education and research, and recognizes the superior achievements of engineers. Dr. Charles M. Vest is president of the National Academy of Engineering.

The **Institute of Medicine** was established in 1970 by the National Academy of Sciences to secure the services of eminent members of appropriate professions in the examination of policy matters pertaining to the health of the public. The Institute acts under the responsibility given to the National Academy of Sciences by its congressional charter to be an adviser to the federal government and, upon its own initiative, to identify issues of medical care, research, and education. Dr. Harvey V. Fineberg is president of the Institute of Medicine.

The **National Research Council** was organized by the National Academy of Sciences in 1916 to associate the broad community of science and technology with the Academy's purposes of furthering knowledge and advising the federal government. Functioning in accordance with general policies determined by the Academy, the Council has become the principal operating agency of both the National Academy of Sciences and the National Academy of Engineering in providing services to the government, the public, and the scientific and engineering communities. The Council is administered jointly by both Academies and the Institute of Medicine. Dr. Ralph J. Cicerone and Dr. Charles M. Vest are chair and vice chair, respectively, of the National Research Council.

www.national-academies.org

COMMITTEE ON OCCUPATIONAL INFORMATION AND ELECTRONIC HEALTH RECORDS

DAVID H. WEGMAN (*Chair*), School of Health and Environment, University of Massachusetts (*Professor Emeritus*)
LAURA O. BRIGHTMAN, Cambridge Health Alliance
CURTIS L. COLE, Weill Cornell Medical College
LETITIA K. DAVIS, Occupational Health Surveillance Program, Massachusetts Department of Public Health
ROBERT A. GREENES, Arizona State University
LAWRENCE HANRAHAN, Wisconsin Division of Public Health
ROBERT HARRISON, University of California, San Francisco
SUNDARESAN JAYARAMAN, Georgia Institute of Technology
MATTHEW KEIFER, Marshfield Clinic Research Foundation
CATHERINE STAES, Biomedical Informatics, University of Utah School of Medicine
GEORGE STAMAS, Division of Occupational Employment Statistics, U.S. Bureau of Labor Statistics

IOM Study Staff
CATHARYN T. LIVERMAN, Project Director
ANDREA M. SCHULTZ, Program Officer
LARISA M. STRAWBRIDGE, Research Associate
JUDITH L. ESTEP, Program Associate

IOM Board on Health Sciences Policy
ANDREW M. POPE, Director

Reviewers

This report has been reviewed in draft form by individuals chosen for their diverse perspectives and technical expertise, in accordance with procedures approved by the National Research Council's Report Review Committee. The purpose of this independent review is to provide candid and critical comments that will assist the institution in making its published report as sound as possible and to ensure that the report meets institutional standards for objectivity, evidence, and responsiveness to the study charge. The review comments and draft manuscript remain confidential to protect the integrity of the deliberative process. We wish to thank the following individuals for their review of this report:

David Bonauto, University of Washington, Seattle
Christopher Chute, Mayo Clinic College of Medicine, Rochester, Minnesota
Carl Kesselman, University of Southern California, Marina del Rey, California
Robert K. McLellan, Dartmouth-Hitchcock Medical Center, Lebanon, New Hampshire
Anna Orlova, Public Health Data Standards Consortium, Baltimore, Maryland
Stephanie L. Reel, Johns Hopkins University, Baltimore, Maryland
Jesse Singer, New York City Department of Health and Mental Hygiene, New York
Walter G. Suarez, Kaiser Permanente, Silver Spring, Maryland
Edward Zuroweste, Migrant Clinicians Network, State College, Pennsylvania

Although the reviewers listed above have provided many constructive comments and suggestions, they were not asked to endorse the conclusions or recommendations, nor did they see the final draft of the report before its release. The review of this report was overseen by **Linda Hawes Clever,** California Pacific Medical Center, San Francisco. Appointed by the Institute of Medicine, she was responsible for making certain that an independent examination of this report was carried out in accordance with institutional procedures and that all review comments were carefully considered. Responsibility for the final content of this report rests entirely with the authoring committee and the institution.

Contents

LETTER TO NIOSH   1

STUDY PROCESS   6

BACKGROUND   7
Occupational Morbidity and Mortality, 7
EHR Use and Incentives for Meaningful Use, 9

BENEFITS OF INCORPORATING OCCUPATIONAL INFORMATION IN THE EHR   11
Improve Quality, Safety, and Efficiency of Care and Reduce Health Disparities, 11
Engage Patients and Families in Their Health Care, 16
Improve Care Coordination, 17
Improve Population and Public Health, 18
Ensure Adequate Privacy and Security Protections for Personal Health Information, 21

FEASIBILITY   22
Current Environment and Technical Considerations for Each Occupational Data Element, 25
Cross-Cutting Challenges and Opportunities, 36
Initial Requirements and Information Modeling, 41

CONCLUSIONS   42

RECOMMENDATIONS 44
Initial Focus on Occupation, Industry, and Work-Relatedness
 Data Elements, 44
Enhance the Value and Use of Occupational Information
 in the EHR, 47

REFERENCES 49

APPENDIXES
A **Workshop Agenda** 59
B **Workshop Participants** 65
C **Committee Biographies** 69

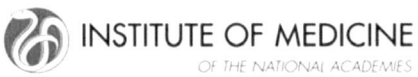

Board on Health Sciences Policy

September 29, 2011

John Howard, M.D.
National Institute for Occupational Safety and Health
Patriots Plaza 1
395 E. Street, S.W., Suite 9200
MS P12
Washington, DC 20201

Dear Dr. Howard:

At the request of the National Institute for Occupational Safety and Health (NIOSH), the Institute of Medicine (IOM) appointed the ad hoc Committee on Occupational Information and Electronic Health Records (EHRs). The overarching charge to the committee was to examine the rationale and feasibility of incorporating occupational information in EHRs and to develop recommendations on next steps for NIOSH and other partners to achieve this goal. More specifically, the committee was asked to analyze the potential benefits of including occupational information in EHRs, examine systems that are currently collecting these data in their EHR in useful ways, and explore the technical challenges that must be overcome in order to facilitate the incorporation of occupational information in EHRs.

Implementation and use of EHRs have increased rapidly since passage of the 2009 Health Information Technology for Economic and Clinical Health (HITECH) Act. The transition from paper to electronic records offers the potential for providing clinicians with relevant and necessary information about their patients' occupations, as well as possibilities for links to an array of clinical decision-support tools that could improve the health care and safety of individuals. Additionally, the inclusion of occupational information in EHRs offers a significant opportunity to advance and expand public health surveillance in order to provide a better understanding of occupational illness and injury. Each year in the United States, more than 4,000 occupational fatalities and more than 3 million occupational injuries occur along with more than 160,000 cases of occupational illnesses (BLS, 2010b, 2011b). Advances in incorporating occupational information in EHRs could lead to more informed clinical diagnosis and treatment plans as well as more effective policies, interventions, and prevention strategies to improve the overall health of the working population.

After gathering and reviewing the available evidence, the committee concluded that occupational information could contribute to fully realizing the meaningful use of EHRs in improving individual and population health care. The report examines the challenges that are inherent in this important advance and makes recommendations (Box 1) focused on moving forward the efforts to incorporate occupational information into EHRs including feasibility studies, demonstration projects, and other actions.

BOX 1
Recommendations

Initial Focus on Occupation, Industry, and Work-Relatedness Data Elements

Recommendation 1: Define the Requirements and Develop Information Models for Storing and Communicating Occupational Information Models for Storing and Communicating Occupational Information and Incorporation of Information on Occupation, Industry, and Work-Relatedness in the EHR
NIOSH, in conjunction with other relevant organizations and initiatives, such as the Public Health Data Standards Consortium and Integrating the Healthcare Enterprise (IHE) International, should conduct demonstration projects involving EHR vendors and health care provider organizations (diverse in the services they provide, populations they serve, and geographic locations) to assess the collection and incorporation of occupation, industry, and work-relatedness data in the EHR at different points in the workflow (including at registration, with the medical assistant, and with the clinician). Further, to examine the bidirectional exchange of occupational data between administrative databases and clinical components in the EHR, NIOSH in conjunction with IHE should conduct an interoperability-testing event (e.g., Connectathon) to demonstrate this bidirectional exchange of occupational information to establish proof of concept and, as appropriate, examine challenges related to variable sources of data and reconciliation of conflicting data.

Recommendation 2: Define the Requirements and Develop Information Models for Storing and Communicating Occupational Information
NIOSH, in conjunction with appropriate domain and informatics experts, should develop new or enhance existing information models for storing occupational information, beginning with occupation, industry, and work-relatedness data and later focusing on employer and exposure data. The information models should consider the various use cases in which the information could be used and use the recommended coding standards. For example, NIOSH should

BOX 1 Continued

consider how best to use social history templates to collect a work history and the problem list to document exposures and abnormal findings and diagnoses with optional work-associated attributes for possible, probable, or definite causes; exposures; and impact on work.

Recommendation 3: <u>Adopt Standard Occupational Classification (SOC) and North American Industry Classification System (NAICS) Coding Standards for Use in the EHR</u>
NIOSH, with assistance from other federal agencies, organizations, and stakeholders (e.g., Bureau of Labor Statistics, Census Bureau, Council of State and Territorial Epidemiologists [CSTE], National Library of Medicine, National Institute of Standards and Technology, National Uniform Billing Committee, Health Level 7 International [HL7]), should recommend to the Health Information Technology (IT) Standards Committee the adoption of SOC and NAICS to code occupation and industry. Furthermore, NIOSH should develop models for reporting health data from EHRs by occupation and industry at different levels of granularity that are meaningful for clinical and public health use.

Recommendation 4: <u>Assess Feasibility of Autocoding Occupational Information Collected in Clinical Settings</u>
NIOSH should place high priority on completing the feasibility assessment of autocoding the narrative information on occupation and, where available, industry that currently is collected and recorded in certain clinical settings, such as the Dartmouth-Hitchcock health care system, Kaiser Permanente, New York State Occupational Health Clinic Network, Cambridge Health Alliance, and hospitals participating in the National Electronic Injury Surveillance System.

Recommendation 5: <u>Develop Meaningful Use Metrics and Performance Measures</u>
Based on findings from the various demonstration projects and feasibility studies, NIOSH, with the assistance of relevant professional organizations and the Health IT Policy Committee, should develop meaningful use metrics and health care performance measures for including occupational information in the meaningful use criteria, beginning with the incorporation of occupation, industry, and work-relatedness data, and later expanding as deemed appropriate to include other data elements such as exposures and employer.

Recommendation 6: <u>Convene a Workshop to Assess Ethical and Privacy Concerns and Challenges Associated with Including Occupational Information in the EHR</u>
NIOSH should convene a workshop involving representatives of labor unions, insurance organizations, health care professional organizations, workers' compensation-related organizations (e.g., International Association of Industrial Accident Boards and Commissions, National Council on Compensation Insurance), and EHR vendors to

Continued

BOX 1 Continued

- assess the implications for the patient and clinician of incorporating work-relatedness in the EHR, with respect to workers' compensation; and
- propose guidelines and policies for protecting the patient's non-work-related health information from inadvertent disclosure and to ensure compliance with the Health Insurance Portability and Accountability Act, workers' compensation, and other privacy standards.

Enhance the Value and Use of Occupational Information in the EHR

Recommendation 7: <u>Develop and Test Innovative Methods for the Collection of Occupational Information for Linking to the EHR</u>
NIOSH should initiate efforts in collaboration with large health care provider organizations, health insurance organizations, EHR vendors, and other stakeholders to develop and test methods for collecting occupational data from innovative sources. Specifically, NIOSH should evaluate collection methods that involve

- patient input through mechanisms such as web-based portals and personal health records, and
- other means such as health-related smart cards, health insurance cards, and human resource systems.

Recommendation 8: <u>Develop Clinical Decision-Support Logic, Education Materials and Return-to-Work Tools</u>
NIOSH, relevant professional organizations, and EHR vendors should begin to develop, test, and iteratively refine and expand

- clinical decision-support tools for common occupational conditions (e.g., work-related asthma);
- tools and programs that could be easily accessed for education of patients and caregivers about occupational illnesses, injuries, and workplace safety;
- training modules for administrative staff to collect occupational information in different care settings; and
- tools to improve and standardize functional job assessment and return-to-work documentation in EHRs, including standards for the transmission of these forms.

Recommendation 9: <u>Develop and Assess Methods for Collecting Standardized Exposure Data</u>
NIOSH should continue to work with occupational and environmental health clinics and other relevant stakeholders to develop and assess methods for collecting standardized exposure data for work-related health conditions. NIOSH should explore the feasibility of

> **BOX 1 Continued**
>
> - listing possible or probable exposures in the problem list or elsewhere in the EHR;
> - linking occupational information in the EHR to online occupational, toxicological, and hazardous materials databases, such as the Occupational Information Network (O*NET), the Association of Occupational and Environmental Clinics, and Haz-Map, to enhance diagnosis and treatment of work-related illnesses and injuries; and
> - automatically generating codes for exposures based on narrative text entries.
>
> Recommendation 10: <u>Assess the Impact of Incorporating Occupational Information in the EHR on Meaningful Use Goals</u>
> NIOSH, in conjunction with relevant stakeholders (e.g., Public Health Data Standards Consortium, CSTE, Association of State and Territorial Health Officials), should
>
> - develop measures and conduct periodic studies to assess the impact of integrating occupational information in EHRs, and
> - estimate the economic impact of EHR-facilitated return-to-work practices for both work-related and non-work-related conditions.

I would like to thank NIOSH and its staff members for supporting this study and for the information they provided to the IOM committee in the course of its work. Appreciation also is due to the IOM committee and staff members for their work in planning the information-gathering workshop that was held in June 2011 and in developing the report and its recommendations. I hope that NIOSH will find this report helpful as it continues to work toward incorporating occupational information in EHRs.

Sincerely,
David H. Wegman, *Chair*
Committee on Occupational Information
and Electronic Health Records

STUDY PROCESS

In early 2011, NIOSH requested that the IOM conduct a study to examine the rationale and feasibility of incorporating occupational[1] information into EHRs and to develop recommendations on next steps for NIOSH and other partners to achieve this goal (see Box 2). This letter report and its recommendations contribute to a larger effort to ensure widespread adoption and meaningful use of EHRs in health care, which has been prompted by incentives that were created by the HITECH Act of 2009.

This study was conducted by the 11-member ad hoc IOM Committee on Occupational Information and Electronic Health Records. The committee included members with expertise in occupational medicine, electronic health records, primary care, public health, biomedical informatics, information technology, and epidemiology (see Appendix C for committee biosketches).

Over the course of the study, the committee held three meetings to gather and review available information, plan and conduct a public workshop, and draft and refine this report's recommendations. The committee's second meeting included a public information-gathering workshop, held June 2, 2011, in Washington, DC (see Appendix A for the workshop agenda and Appendix B for a list of registered attendees). The workshop provided the committee with insights from experts in primary care, occupational medicine, public health surveillance, and information technology. Presentations and discussion focused on the potential benefits and challenges of including occupational information in EHRs to improve health care delivery and public health surveillance, the extent to which and the manner in which this information is currently being recorded in EHRs, and technical considerations related to standardizing and maximizing the value of the data. Additional information on occupational morbidity and mortality, as well as on EHRs and meaningful use, was collected in a literature search and reviewed by the committee to inform its deliberations.

---

[1] Throughout this report, "occupational" is used broadly to describe attributes related to one's occupation (e.g., secretary), industry (e.g., mining), employer (e.g., Ford), and work environment (e.g., exposure to asbestos). Occupational illness, injury, and fatalities are used to denote morbidity and mortality related to employment and work environment.

> **BOX 2**
> **Statement of Task**
>
> At the request of the National Institute for Occupational Safety and Health (NIOSH), the Institute of Medicine (IOM) will conduct a study to examine the rationale and feasibility of incorporating work history information into patient electronic health records. NIOSH seeks to ensure meaningful use of occupational information in electronic health records by 2015. This will require the agency's demonstration of feasibility by 2013.
>
> An ad hoc committee will plan and hold data-gathering meetings, including a public workshop; conduct analysis; hold deliberations; and prepare a letter report with findings and recommendations that will address the following issues:
>
> - Significance—What are the potential benefits to individual and public health of incorporating occupational information in electronic health records?
> - Current environment—Are there current systems which incorporate work history into the record in a manner which supports clinical decision making and public health reporting activities?
> - Technical issues—What are the perceived technical barriers to incorporating work history information into the patient's electronic health record? What are the barriers to using current systems of coding industry and occupation? What are alternatives to current methods? How would the technical issues be best addressed by electronic health record system vendors and researchers?
> - Next steps—What steps are needed to advance this effort? What efforts by NIOSH in conjunction with government and non-governmental partners are needed?

BACKGROUND

Occupational Morbidity and Mortality

Employed Americans spend almost half of their waking hours at work (BLS, 2011a). The nature of the work environment and work tasks can have a significant impact on workers' health and even on the health of family members. Physical, chemical, radiological, biological, and ergonomic hazards can cause injury and illness, as can organizational attributes of the workplace, such as stress and other psychosocial factors. The work environment can also influence personal lifestyle choices. Health care professionals need to understand their patients' work environment in order to diagnose and treat certain illnesses and injuries and to recommend medical restrictions or work environment modifications that will help them recover and prevent additional harm. Identification and documentation of work-related health problems by health care professionals can also lead to interventions that protect other workers at risk.

Work demands can contribute to common health problems not generally associated with employment. For example, Church and colleagues (2011) suggested that decreasing energy expenditures at work over the last 50 years could explain a significant portion of Americans' increase in body weight. On the other hand, the workplace can offer health promotion and disease prevention benefits, including wellness programs (e.g., stress reduction classes, smoking cessation programs) and facilities (e.g., exercise rooms). These types of programs have been demonstrated to be successful when interventions for behavior change occur in the workplace (Okechukwu et al., 2009; Sorensen et al., 2009, 2010).

U.S. estimates of the annual number of nonfatal injuries at work range from 3.1 million to 5.5 million (BLS, 2010b; Schulte, 2005; Smith et al., 2005), with more than 3 million of these leading to at least a partial day out of work (Smith et al., 2005). The Bureau of Labor Statistics (BLS) reported 4,547 deaths in 2010 due to occupational injury (BLS, 2011b).[2] BLS (2010b) estimates the annual number of acute occupational illnesses to be about 166,000.

Steenland and colleagues (2003) estimate more than 55,000 U.S. occupational deaths per year, including 6,200 from injuries and 49,000 from known occupational illnesses, making occupational causes the nation's eighth leading cause of death. An estimated 15 percent of asthma deaths, 14 percent of deaths due to chronic obstructive pulmonary disease, and 2.4 to 4.8 percent of all cancer deaths are attributable to occupational exposures (Steenland et al., 2003).

The costs of occupational injuries, illnesses, and deaths are high. In 2008, employers paid $78.9 billion in workers' compensation premiums (Sengupta et al., 2010). The overall costs to workers and their employers, when taking into account direct health care costs and indirect costs, such as lost productivity, range from $128 billion to $170 billion per year (Schulte, 2005; Thomsen et al., 2007).

The current surveillance systems for occupational health, including BLS and workers' compensation databases, do not fully capture the impact of occupational injuries and illnesses (GAO, 2009). The BLS Survey of Occupational Injuries and Illnesses (SOII) derives its non-fatal

---

[2] The Census of Fatal Occupational Injuries, conducted by the BLS, integrates data from 25 sources (e.g., death certificates, government agency administrative reports, the Current Population Survey) to estimate mortality due to occupational injury.

workplace injury and illness data from a sample of Occupational Safety and Health Administration (OSHA) logs kept by employers, which enable estimates across states. The SOII undercounts occupational injuries and illnesses for several reasons, including scope (e.g., these estimates do not cover self-employed workers, federal government employees, and others) and delayed recognition of cases, including those with long latency periods (Boden et al., 2010; GAO, 2009; Hilaski, 1981; Oleinick and Zaidman, 2010; Rosenman et al., 2006). Less severe conditions, requiring workers to miss less than a week of work, also have a lower probability of being recorded (Boden et al., 2010).

A key factor that contributes to underreporting of occupational morbidity, particularly illnesses, is that reporting relies on the health care professional's recognition of a health condition as work related.[3] Many such connections are overlooked or misdiagnosed (Landrigan and Baker, 1991; Steenland et al., 2003) and thus go unreported or are misclassified. This is especially true for chronic conditions and diseases with a long latency period, such as many types of cancer (Ruser, 2008; Souza et al., 2010a).

For any number of reasons, patients may not suggest to their clinician that an injury or illness may be work related. They may not be aware that they could be eligible for workers' compensation or the benefits may be too small to warrant the time and effort to report a minor problem (Azaroff et al., 2002; Fan et al., 2006). They may fear employer retaliation or stigma if they report health problems (Azaroff et al., 2002; Boden and Ozonoff, 2008; Boden et al., 2010; Fan et al., 2006). Employers that offer incentives based on the length of time without injuries may create incentives not to report (Azaroff et al., 2002). Employers also have incentives to avoid reporting: high injury rates may result in a loss of business, more frequent OSHA inspections, or high workers' compensation insurance rates (Azaroff et al., 2002; Boden et al., 2010).

EHR Use and Incentives for Meaningful Use

The transition to EHRs is moving ahead rapidly. Health care provider organizations (primary care and specialist physician offices, hospitals, health systems, specialty clinics, and community and public health clinics) are in the midst of adopting new EHR systems, and health care pro-

---

[3]Throughout this report, "work related" is used to denote caused by or aggravated by work (WHO Expert Committee, 1985).

fessionals and staff are establishing habits of working with the new systems. The percentage of office-based physicians with basic EHR capability rose from 11 percent in 2006 to an estimated 21 percent in 2009 (ONC, 2010). In 2008, 8 percent of U.S. hospitals reported having basic EHR capability (ONC, 2010).

Driving EHR development and providing financial incentives for implementation is the HITECH Act of 2009. The Act provides funds to the Office of the National Coordinator for Health Information Technology (ONC) to promote the implementation of health information technology and an estimated $27 billion for the Centers for Medicare and Medicaid Services (CMS) to use as incentive payments for physician's offices and hospitals to support adoption of EHRs[4] (CMS, 2010b). The incentives require that providers use a certified EHR product and fulfill a set of objectives that demonstrate "meaningful use" of EHRs.[5] ONC has detailed a set of certification criteria for EHRs that stipulate the technical capabilities required to ensure data security, confidentiality, interoperability, and capability to perform specific functions. Its EHR certification process is conducted by private-sector organizations approved as ONC-Authorized Testing and Certification Bodies (HHS, 2010). Hospitals that are not using certified EHRs according to meaningful use criteria by 2015 will face reduced reimbursements.

Several of the Stage 1 objectives are particularly relevant to the inclusion of occupational information in EHRs, including the requirement that electronic records "maintain up-to-date problem list of current and active diagnoses," "use certified EHR technology to identify patient-specific education resources and provide those resources to the patient, if appropriate," and have the "capability to submit electronic data on reportable (as required by state or local law) lab results to public health agencies and actual submission in accordance with applicable law and practice" (CMS, 2010c).

---

[4] Health care professionals who do not see Medicare or Medicaid patients are not eligible for the CMS incentives (CMS, 2010a).

[5] ONC expects to implement the meaningful use requirements in three stages (42 CFR 412, 413, 422, and 495). The first stage was released in July 2010 (45 CFR 170) and focuses on EHR functionality, including data capture. For Stage 1, the maximum incentive per eligible health care provider is $18,000; for hospitals, the base incentive payment is $2 million (CMS, 2010a). Although the timelines are somewhat flexible, Stage 2 implementation is anticipated for 2013 (CMS, 2011) and is expected to focus on structured health information exchange (42 CFR 412, 413, 422, and 495). Stage 3 implementation is anticipated for 2015 (CMS, 2011) and is expected to focus on patient-centered health information exchange and clinical decision support (42 CFR 412, 413, 422, and 495).

BENEFITS OF INCORPORATING OCCUPATIONAL INFORMATION IN THE EHR

As part of its statement of task, the committee was asked to respond to the question: What are the potential benefits to individual and public health of incorporating occupational information in electronic health records? The committee organized its response around the five health care outcomes and policy priorities used to categorize the Stage 1 "meaningful use" objectives (CMS, 2010c):

1. Improve the quality, safety, and efficiency of care and reduce health disparities.
2. Engage patients and families in their health care.
3. Improve care coordination.
4. Improve population and public health.
5. Ensure adequate privacy and security protections for personal health information.

In responding to the second part of the task on technical feasibility, the committee decided to examine the individual occupational data elements that are commonly used in occupational health data collection and are considered the most useful for clinical and public health purposes—occupation, industry, work-relatedness, employer, and exposures. The committee also explored the steps, such as information modeling, that need to occur to provide detailed specifications for each of the data elements. These data elements are defined and described in depth later in the report, but they are introduced here to provide context for the following section, which outlines a number of potential benefits of incorporating occupational information in EHRs.

Improve Quality, Safety, and Efficiency of Care and Reduce Health Disparities

Providing occupational information to the clinician could increase the likelihood of arriving at a correct diagnosis and improve the management, treatment, and return to work of patients, regardless of the etiology of their health condition. Several examples of the potential benefits were presented and discussed at the IOM's June 2011 workshop (Box 3).

> **BOX 3**
> **Examples of the Value of Occupational Information**
> **for Diagnosis and Clinical Care**
>
> Workshop participants provided examples of how knowing a person's occupation and industry might assist health care professionals in identifying the cause of an illness and enabling more efficient and effective care. These examples fall into three main categories:
>
> 1. Inform diagnosis for
>   - workers exposed to respiratory hazards (e.g., occupational asthma),
>   - workers who handle chemicals (e.g., occupational dermatitis), and
>   - older workers exposed to noise (e.g., hearing loss wrongly attributed to age).
>
> 2. Improve treatment and inform plans for return to work by understanding
>   - the impact of shift work and irregular schedules (e.g., exacerbations of diabetes),
>   - legal requirements for return to normal duties (e.g., commercial drivers who have had a heart attack),
>   - choice of non-drowsy medications for people who work with heavy machinery,
>   - the need to keep food handlers out of work until they are noninfectious, and
>   - choice of high blood pressure medications (e.g., diuretics) for people working in hot environments.
>
> 3. Provide education opportunities and connections to wellness programs such as
>   - links to websites, printouts, or other educational materials in multiple languages;
>   - community (i.e., non-employer) resources for workers; and
>   - integration of occupational and clinical health records and links to employer resources (e.g., employee assistance programs, health coaching, workability programs), community primary care, and other resources.
>
> SOURCES: McLellan, 2011; Tacci, 2011; Wagner, 2011; Zuroweste, 2011.

Facilitate and Inform Clinical Diagnoses and Treatment

Inclusion of information in the EHR about the type of work that patients do could enable more accurate diagnosis and treatment of a number of medical problems, thereby improving both the quality and the efficiency of care. Currently, clinicians might not consider work exposure in the etiology of a patient's illness until after a lengthy, inefficient, trial-and-error period. Available occupational information could lead health care professionals to consider the potential occupational hazards (e.g., chemical, biomechanical, physical, biological, psychological) and stresses (e.g., shift work, long hours) that might impact or be impacted by health conditions. Some work-related conditions are relatively rare, and new chemicals and processes are constantly being introduced into workplaces. When clinicians are aware that their patients have an ongoing occupational exposure to specific, potentially harmful agents, they can monitor signs and symptoms and obtain appropriate laboratory tests for early detection of harmful effects. Having access to a worker's occupational data may also be helpful in informing the clinician's understanding of possible exposures to reproductive hazards. Further, given that children may accompany their parents to their workplace or may be exposed to toxins (e.g., on their parents' clothing), the collection of parents' occupational information may also enable improved diagnoses of health conditions in children who have paraoccupational exposures.

Occupational exposures can be important risk factors for chronic diseases such as cancer. For example, workers exposed to benzene or benzene-containing solvents, commonly used in the 1960s, are at risk of developing acute myeloid leukemia later in life; acute myeloid leukemia resulting from benzene exposure has an average latency period of 12 years (Haz-Map, 2011). By the time actual disease develops, an exposed person may have changed jobs or retired. A list of a person's jobs could be collected over time in the EHR, creating an occupational history that, if easily searchable, could provide important clues to these past exposures, the specific characteristics of the resultant disease, and its appropriate treatment.

Develop Appropriate Recovery and Return-to-Work Plans

Knowledge about the occupational environment may improve the management of patients' conditions and the quality and efficiency of care, regardless of the etiology of the health problem (Tacci, 2011). For example, patients with diabetes who work night shifts may need a treatment plan that includes additional monitoring, since irregular hours tend to disrupt insulin management.

Many occupational health problems do not present with signs or symptoms that differ from non-work-related health problems. For example, low back pain occurs in approximately two-thirds of U.S. adults at some point in life (Lawrence et al., 2008), and an estimated 65 percent of back pain cases result from acute or cumulative trauma at work (Guo et al., 1995). Accurate occupational information in the EHR would help clarify the worksite's role in the injury and illness and enable clinicians to devise a recovery plan that accommodates job demands—an essential factor in rehabilitation and in the development of appropriate return-to-work plans.

Health care professionals who understand their patients' work demands and occupational environment can draw attention to specific steps needed to minimize or eliminate hazards and increase the safety of the individual and, perhaps, other workers. For example, analysis and correction of ergonomic hazards may prevent recurrence of musculoskeletal disorders, allowing employees to recover and return to work more quickly. If the correction of such hazards becomes institutionalized throughout the workplace, similar injuries and exacerbations could be prevented in other employees.

Facilitate the Workers' Compensation Process

To receive medical and indemnity payments related to temporary or permanent work-related disability, employees must file for workers' compensation benefits with their employer, and their clinician must submit notification of treatment to the workers' compensation insurance carrier. Efficient, effective, and prompt treatment for an occupationally related health condition improves quality of care, yet often depends on timely notification of the workers' compensation program, which an EHR can facilitate or, perhaps, automate. The National Committee on Vital and Health Statistics and other organizations are charged by the Patient Protection and Affordable Care Act of 2010 to explore this issue and examine whether or not standards and operating rules should apply to workers' compensation transactions (H.R. 3590 Section 10109 (b)(2)).

Increase Use of Treatment Guidelines and Adherence to Safety Standards

When the diagnosis of an occupational illness or injury is made, the EHR could guide clinicians to additional information and clinical decision support, as well as to reporting requirements and quality metrics to ensure that care conforms to recommended treatment guidelines such as those promulgated by several state workers' compensation systems and various authoritative medical organizations.[6] Decision-support tools could link clinicians to appropriate web-based guidelines on occupational illnesses and injuries, including resources related to exposures, occupational tasks, or occupational specialists.

A number of workplace safety standards require medical monitoring of people exposed to specific hazards, such as lead and asbestos, and occupational data in the EHR could help assure ongoing clinical management of workers exposed to these types of hazards. Additionally, occupational information in the EHR could have safety benefits during the course of medical treatment both for individual patients and for their coworkers. For the individual, quicker diagnosis of an occupational illness reduces the risks of unnecessary diagnostic testing; all employees benefit from timely hazard remediation.

Reduce Health Disparities

Low-income, immigrant, and minority workers may be at disproportionate risk from occupational hazards, because they are more likely to be employed in high-risk jobs or in workplaces where hazards are not adequately controlled (McCauley, 2005; RWJF, 2008). A number of additional factors can contribute to occupational health disparities among racial, ethnic, and socioeconomic groups. Because low-income and marginal workers face challenges to their economic security, they may hesitate to speak up about occupational safety concerns for fear of losing their jobs. They may have less knowledge about occupational risks and safety standards. Workplace discrimination, unequal access to health care professionals with occupational health training, and literacy, language, or other communication barriers can also contribute to these disparities (Souza et al., 2010b).

Documentation of health disparities is an important step in responding to these problems. The routine inclusion of occupational information in the health history could encourage hesitant workers to voice concerns to their primary care provider in a less threatening context. Additionally, prompting clinicians to seek information on occupation could allow for improved documentation of disparities in occupational health risks, and this information can provide the basis for targeted interventions to improve quality of and access to care. Furthermore, there has been some

---

[6]For example, Colorado Department of Labor and Employment, 2011; New York State Workers' Compensation Board, 2010; Washington State Department of Labor and Industries, 2011.

research on the correlation between low job status and poor health status; for example, Clougherty and colleagues (2010) found that blue-collar workers had an elevated risk for hypertension in comparison to white-collar workers. The ability to establish causality and further explore the influence of work on health, particularly as it may affect workers with poorer health status, could be facilitated by the inclusion of occupational information in the EHR. Information about occupational health disparities may also foster integrated approaches to manage and care for the health needs of vulnerable populations that take into account interacting factors at work, at home, and in the community.

Engage Patients and Families in Their Health Care

Provide Educational Resources

Incorporating occupational information in EHRs could provide opportunities to educate patients and families about occupational risks and prevention strategies and could link patients with available services provided by employers, as well as other community organizations. For example, information about hazards and prevention strategies could be provided to patients diagnosed with common occupational health conditions (e.g., tendinitis, dermatitis) and to patients exposed to hazards in common occupations and industries (e.g., sun exposure in agricultural workers, silica exposures in construction, burn hazards in food service).

While prevention information is usually targeted toward the person seeking care, occupational information could also enable prevention efforts that target others, such as reducing prenatal exposure risks for a worker's pregnant spouse or hazardous exposures for household members who may be exposed to toxins (lead, pesticides) brought home on the worker's clothing.

Link Patients with Other Services

Knowing who a patient's employer is and having access to information about the employer's health promotion programs could allow clinicians to link patients to these resources, regardless of the etiology of their condition.

Although this report is focused on the EHR, a growing number of Americans also have personal health records (PHRs), which may allow them to track and/or enter data online regarding their health history, immunizations, and health promotion activities, as well as gain access to health promotion information resources such as those mentioned above (Archer et al., 2011). Some PHRs are hosted by health care systems and provider organizations (so-called tethered PHRs) and provide access to information in the EHR or exchange of certain information between the PHR and the EHR. The PHR is a potential source of occupational information for the EHR and could serve as a means of communication, education, and even decision support for patients regarding occupational injury, illness, risk, and prevention. Sharing of health-related data could be improved through smart card technologies that allow easy transport of a patient's medical record and health history between health care professionals and that provide access to information on prescriptions, insurance, and reimbursements. This technology is in use in several European and Asian countries and under exploration in others. Overcoming challenges including those associated with data privacy, security, and standardization is key to the implementation of this type of technology (Frost and Sullivan, 2010; Hsu et al., 2011; Kliff, 2010).

Improve Care Coordination

Advise Clinicians of Applicable Occupational Information

As patients move through the health care system, their occupational information may help each of the many clinicians they encounter to provide better, more coordinated care. Effective communication and coordinated approaches across health care professionals—such as hospital staff, primary care practitioners, specialists, occupational and physical therapists, complementary health practitioners, and mental health professionals—should focus on preparing the person to attain maximum function, including returning to work, if applicable. Currently, not all of these professional groups are adequately prepared to assess and manage conditions from the return-to-work perspective.

A review of return-to-work notes provided to Kaiser Permanente's health plan members showed that clinicians, depending on their specialty, provided assessments of temporary total disability at widely varying rates for the same condition. Education about "reducing variance" trimmed excessive temporary total disability assessments by 10 to 30 percent (Papanek, 2011). Before the educational intervention, primary care physicians and orthopedists gave a temporary total disability work note for ankle sprains and low back pain 50 to 80 percent of the time, whereas occupational medicine clinicians gave one only 10 to 20 percent of the time. Keeping people on the job or returning them to work as rapidly as possible is clinically important, in part because people with low back pain may avoid activities they are capable of doing because of fear of injury (Crombez et al., 1999).

Integrate Occupational and General Health Information

A standardized approach to collecting occupational information could improve communication and coordination among all users of the EHR. At present, this information (if available) is often dispersed across multiple paper and electronic record systems maintained by general or specialty health care professionals, administrative offices of health care professionals, non-employer-based occupational health clinics, individuals in their PHRs, personnel or human resource departments, and employee health records (if the person has consented to have it included). Even within EHRs, occupational information can be entered in various sections (e.g., demographics, social history, medical notes, the problem list). Integrating occupational information in the EHR could bring together relevant data while also requiring appropriate "firewalls" or other security measures that could ensure patient privacy and comply with the Health Insurance Portability and Accountability Act (HIPAA) and workers' compensation regulations (discussed further in the section on privacy protections).

Improve Population and Public Health

The true burden of work-related illnesses, injuries, and deaths is difficult to determine; as noted above, available public health surveillance systems and data sources are not comprehensive in scope, and, for various reasons, workers and employers may be reluctant to report. These obstacles limit the ability of public health programs to most effectively target interventions to protect workers. The inclusion of occupational information in EHRs presents an opportunity to improve all core public health functions—assessment, policy development, and assurance of services (IOM, 1988)—by enabling more complete surveillance and improvements in disease and injury prevention policies and programs based on surveillance findings.

Improve Public Health Reporting and Surveillance

When patients are diagnosed with specific communicable diseases (e.g., as infections with *salmonella*, hepatitis A, measles, tuberculosis), health care professionals are required to report the case to public health authorities. Public health authorities then investigate the source of infection so as to prevent further transmission. Knowledge of a patient's workplace and occupation is essential in assessing transmission risks and often in implementing mitigation and preventive measures. As examples, a food handler or child care worker with *salmonella* poses an acute risk, and a customer service agent who comes in contact with many people poses more risk than someone who works from home.

Among the nationally notifiable infectious conditions, information is often collected in the initial case report in order to prioritize and plan a public health response. For example, the majority of California's infectious disease case report forms require occupation as a separate line item (California Department of Public Health, 2010). Despite its importance, current infectious disease reporting is known to be incomplete, depending on the seriousness of the illness and the resources devoted to its treatment and prevention (Doyle et al., 2002). EHRs raise the possibility of automated and more systematic reporting that could include vital occupational information.

In many states, health care professionals are required to report certain work-related health conditions (e.g., silicosis, work-related asthma, elevated lead levels, serious injuries) to the state health department for surveillance purposes and potential public health intervention. Such reports require sufficient information to ensure appropriate investigation or implementation of public health measures. Similarly, employers are required to report specific conditions and injuries to OSHA or workers' compensation programs. For various reasons, clinicians and employers alike underreport these problems (Pransky et al., 1999; Swotinsky, 2009). To the extent that health care professionals do not report because they are unaware of the requirement or because the reporting process is too cumbersome, EHRs could include reminders or make the reporting automatic—and thereby improve the quality of surveillance and the timeliness of potential public health responses (Overhage et al., 2008; Silk and Berkelman, 2005; Staes et al., 2009; Ward et al., 2005). Additionally, because there is no current uniform format or standard for the secure collection, storage, transmission, and use of patient information for public health case reporting, it is difficult to harness data from various sources for research and public health policy. Having this information available in a standard electronic format offers the potential for improved public health surveillance of reportable conditions, research, and response.

More broadly, systematic inclusion of occupational information in EHRs could overcome some of the limitations of current occupational injury and illness surveillance systems that rely heavily on employer reporting and cover limited populations and conditions. Inclusion of occupational information in EHRs would allow population-based surveillance of work-related illness and injury, providing information about trends that could inform priorities for policy, educational, and technological interventions to reduce the burden of occupational disease and injury. The data could be used to assess progress in meeting both prevention and health care quality goals. In addition to conducting public health surveillance at national and state levels, these data could also be useful when surveillance is conducted at the community or accountable care organization levels to guide targeted community health initiatives to promote healthy living among the population served. As noted, the data may also be used to document disparities in occupational risks that can be the basis of interventions to improve health equity.

Incorporation of occupational information in EHRs may also provide data that could be used for epidemiologic and biomedical research to describe and identify new associations between work and health. Furthermore, the collection of occupational health information could help inform other public health efforts, such as vital records, disease registries, health policy studies, and environmental public health efforts. Often a first step in assessing the environmental cause of a community disease cluster is to rule out occupational exposures.

Improve Community and Preventive Services

The workplace is increasingly recognized as a venue for reaching populations to promote healthy living, and working conditions themselves can influence lifestyle choices and personal behavior. Aggregated EHR data could serve as the evidence base for establishing workplace wellness programs. With consistent and accurate data, aggregate population health statistics could be calculated by employer, industry sector, and occupation, in order to benchmark health care costs and quality, target health promotion efforts, and assess wellness program results. For example, the prevalence of smoking by occupation can inform the development of smoking policies as well as the provision of smoking cessation programs for occupational groups (National Survey on Drug Use and Health, 2009), taking advantage of the strength of social networks.

Integrated approaches that take into account occupational risk factors have potential for improving health behaviors (Sorensen et al., 2009, 2010). Likewise, information about obesity by occupation could foster development of integrated approaches to healthy living that account for the influence of both working conditions and lifestyle choices. Incorporating occupational information in EHRs could have additional benefits such as triggering decision support and monitoring the quality of recommended preventive services for at-risk groups, such as increasing the proportion of adults "who have discussed with a . . . health professional whether their asthma was work related," a Healthy People 2020 developmental objective (Healthy People 2020, 2010, p. 6).

Identify New Occupational Illnesses

Clusters of patients with similar signs, symptoms, and work histories are often the first signal of a new or emerging occupational illness (Kreiss, 2011; Luckhaupt et al., 2011). For example, information about patients' employment was critical for making the link between severe obstructive lung disease and exposure to the chemical diacetyl used in food flavorings (NIOSH, 2004). However, such associations currently depend on either an astute clinician who happens to see several such cases and makes a link or an employee's report of several coworkers with similar conditions. Systematic documentation of employer name, industry, and employee occupation in an EHR could facilitate the identification and investigation of clusters.

Ensure Adequate Privacy and Security Protections for Personal Health Information

Information relevant to a patient's work (e.g., employer, occupation, industry) is often collected for billing and for recording the individual's background or history and is protected by standard HIPAA regulations (P.L. 104-191). Other occupational information, such as employee medical records or links between the patient's diagnosis and work, may have to be sequestered through firewalls or other security measures in the EHR system, as part of OSHA medical record keeping standards (29 CFR 1910.1020) or workers' compensation program requirements, so as to limit who can access that information. The need to establish firewalls and other security measures is not unique to occupational information. In addition to HIPAA privacy rules on "protected health information," a number of other federal laws are relevant to health privacy. The Americans with Disabilities Act (ADA) (P.L. 110-325) and Genetic Information Nondiscrimination Act (H.R. 493) generally require employers to keep medical information confidential and make it illegal for them to use this information for decisions related to employment terms, including hiring, promoting, or firing.

With the advent of the EHR, new standards for Health Information Exchange (HIE) are being developed explicitly to facilitate care coordination via the exchange of data among health care professionals.[7] However, the optimal HIE mechanisms for occupational health data have not yet been determined. As EHRs continue to be refined and to incorporate processes that have been handled through multiple paper files, the integration of these data will involve protecting confidentiality while also allowing for coordination of care when appropriate and necessary. Because these rules and regulations are frequently changing and vary by location and setting, firewalls and other security measures need to be flexible.

FEASIBILITY

Bearing these potential benefits of EHRs in mind, the committee considered the feasibility of getting occupational information into and out of the EHR most efficiently to improve clinical care and public health efforts. For each of the occupational data elements that are commonly used in occupational health data collection and that could potentially be included in the EHR (i.e., occupation, industry, work-relatedness, employer, and exposures), the committee examined the current environment as well as the technical considerations that would have to be explored to achieve the anticipated benefits. The committee reviewed challenges and opportunities associated with the collection and

---

[7] For example, HL7's Continuity of Care Document and Clinical Document Architecture (Dolin et al., 2006; HL7, 2007).

use of occupational data, as well as the need for a standardized information model. The committee's assessments were informed by the workshop presentations and discussions with users of EHR systems in primary care and occupational and environmental health clinics that currently incorporate occupational information into patient records (see Box 4). Additionally, the workshop highlighted the range of existing regulations that require reporting to various entities such as workers' compensation divisions and CMS. EHRs developed with these needs in mind can enable facilitated and structured reporting while ensuring privacy protections. Further examination of the regulatory reporting environment is needed but was beyond the scope of this letter report.

BOX 4
Examples of Collecting and Using Occupational Information in EHRs

Primary Care

Cambridge Health Alliance (CHA) Primary Care Clinics Pilot Project (Personal communication, L. Brightman [Cambridge Health Alliance] and T. Davis [Massachusetts Department of Public Health], August 3, 2011)

- The aim of the pilot, which was conducted in collaboration with the Massachusetts Department of Public Health and funded by NIOSH, was to increase the capacity of the clinic to identify and meet the occupational health needs of patients and to improve surveillance of their conditions.
- Information about patient occupation was collected and entered at registration by trained registrars. In the EHR, occupation and employer information entered during registration appeared in the demographic section of the EHR as well as in the social history section, where the clinician could enter additional free text information.
- The problem list section of the EHR included an option for the clinician to classify a health problem as suspected to be work related.
- Patient and health care professional education materials about occupational health conditions were included on the CHA intranet, which is available to clinicians.
- Follow-up efforts are assessing the feasibility of assigning standard codes to the more than 20,000 occupation titles collected during 2010 using the NIOSH automated coding system that is in development.

Continued

BOX 4 Continued

Occupational and Environmental Health Services

Dartmouth-Hitchcock (D-H) Medical Center (McLellan, 2011)

- The D-H Medical Center developed an Employee Report of Injury (EROI) form and process, which is housed online on the D-H intranet and available offsite through a virtual private network. The report can be filled out by the employee or the supervisor to report an occupational injury or illness.
- The EROI sends an automatic e-mail alert to appropriate departments (e.g., occupational medicine, safety, human resources).
- The EROI interfaces with the human resources database and is automatically populated with occupation-related data (e.g., job title, department, supervisor, shift, hours worked, employment status). These data link to an internal database with information on job demands and exposures. In the future, the EROI will be linked to the Occupational Information Network (O*NET), a Department of Labor-funded program that surveys workers to determine their occupation and includes an application that can be freely searched online (National Center for O*NET Development, 2011).
- The EROI also interfaces with the D-H occupational health EHR, where it automatically populates OSHA and workers' compensation reporting forms. The occupational health EHR can be tracked by different variables (e.g., workgroup, shift, supervisor, job type) to assess population health.
- The EROI has led to increased reporting. Since its implementation, the number of reports of injury has more than doubled.

Kaiser Permanente (Papanek, 2011)

- Kaiser has developed an Occupational Medicine EHR that includes a module on work restrictions and disability documentation.
- Still to come are functions that can produce legally mandated workers' compensation or other reports and secure communication for external stakeholders (e.g., employers, insurers, public health agencies).

Long Island Occupational and Environmental Health Center (LIOEHC) (Cocchiarella, 2011)

- The LIOEHC is developing an EHR called E*Healthline, which includes patient and employer screens and portals.
- During an in-person visit to the LIOEHC, the patient answers five questions related to industry and occupation that are reviewed by the health care professional. Within E*Healthline, a dropdown box provides the appropriate industry code for the entered description of industry, and the job title and description can be imported.

BOX 4 Continued

- Entering a sentinel diagnosis or exposure prompts decision support for the health care professional, including management and treatment guidelines.
- E*Healthline will automatically populate forms the patient needs for workers' compensation, return to work, and disability assessment.

Current Environment and Technical Considerations for Each Occupational Data Element

Occupation

The data element "occupation" asks for the individual's job title, although a general description of a person's work may also be included. Being asked one's occupation is a familiar question to many people because it is asked on commonly completed forms and surveys. Having information on a patient's occupation in the EHR can raise the clinician's awareness that work exposures or conditions should be considered in diagnosis or treatment decisions and can prompt education about occupational risks. Box 5 illustrates the use of data on occupation as well as the other potential data elements.

Current environment Occupation is a construct widely used as a proxy for hazardous work exposures in clinical settings as well as in occupational health and safety surveillance and research. Occupation is collected in research studies and by many national health and economic surveys,[8] and standard questions and training tools for surveyors have been developed and tested. The applicability of these questions and tools to the clinical setting remains to be evaluated.

As noted above, many states request occupation as a data element in reports of occupational diseases. Usual occupation is collected on the standard death certificate (NCHS, 2003) and is required to be reported, if available, in the medical record sent to state cancer registries (NAACCR, 2011). Collection of occupation (and industry) in the uniform bill re-

---

[8]Surveys that record occupation include the American Community Survey, the Current Population Survey, the National Health Interview Survey, the Occupational Employment Statistics Survey, and the Survey of Occupational Injuries and Illnesses.

quired by CMS and private insurers is currently under consideration (Taylor, 2011).

In the health care environment, a data element for occupation is included in most medical registration systems for administrative and reimbursement purposes, but the information, if collected, is rarely integrated with clinical data. Within EHRs, occupation may be recorded in a variety of places and formats, which limits its potential usefulness in queries or searches, decision support, and public health reporting. For example, a patient's occupation may be entered as narrative text documented in clinical notes or in social history templates, occupation fields, or other templates developed for specific purposes.

For a number of facilities in the Cambridge Health Alliance, a large Massachusetts health care system, occupation is collected in the administrative record and auto-populates the clinical section of the EHR (see Box 4). The registrar documents a single occupation and this becomes part of the social history in the clinical record where the clinician can add additional information about current or past occupations. In this system, occupational data do not flow bi-directionally between the registration and clinical components so these clinical updates do not change the administrative record. Reports can only be run off the occupation field in the administrative record, which does not include the clinical updates (Personal communication, Laura Brightman, Cambridge Health Alliance, August 1, 2011).

Strategies to code narrative text data on occupation are improving. NIOSH is currently testing and enhancing an autocoder application that can automatically assign standard occupation and industry codes from narrative text (NIOSH, 2011a). Preliminary tests of the autocoding tool suggest approximately a 70 percent success rate for autocoding free text with about 90 percent of these being accurately translated when compared to manual coding (NIOSH, 2011b). Industry information is used in assigning some, but not all, occupation codes. It would be useful for NIOSH to assess the extent to which the data element for industry is needed to accurately code occupation before making a final determination about the need to collect industry as well as occupation in the EHR.

Technical considerations While the job title alone does not reveal specific exposures, it can suggest common risks, prompt the clinician to ask for details on exposures and work conditions, and provide access to clinical decision-support tools. Currently, clinical decision-support tools are often nonstandard and vendor-specific, but over time they may become standardized.

To be most useful, especially for public health surveillance and research purposes, data on occupation need to be standardized. Most of the examples reviewed by the committee use the BLS's Standard Occupational Classification (SOC) system or the U.S. Census Bureau's occupation codes, which are derived from the SOC.[9] Collection and coding of occupation must balance the level of detail requested with the individual's or employer's ability to report these data.

Data on occupation may be collected directly from the patient. As noted above, the autocoder technology that assigns standardized codes from narrative text is being further refined, and the integration of an autocoder into EHR or PHR systems, which could potentially retrieve information from external applications, eventually might be feasible. In the long term, the standardization of open source autocoder services or content should be considered to enable the generation of comparable and consistent information. To add additional information on specific occupations, use of the Occupational Information Network (O*NET) database could be explored since this resource provides occupation-specific information using SOC codes (National Center for O*NET Development, 2011).

Human resources or payroll systems could be additional potential sources of data on occupation for health care systems serving large employers. Employer-specific job titles or codes would have to be crosswalked to the SOC codes, which could be a challenge because employers often use variable or employer-specific terms. Provider organizations experimenting with EHRs might attempt to integrate data on occupation from their own human resources departments, as both a compelling example and a way to work out potential problems. The Dartmouth-Hitchcock system has done this for its 9,000 employees and their 9,700 dependents (McLellan, 2011).

The EHR, which can be used to follow individuals over time and across employers, can maintain an occupational history. Relevant work history information can be built over time by updating current occupation at each health care encounter or on a regular basis. "Usual" occupation, which is generally defined as the longest-held job, could be derived from the history. For people who are retired or unemployed it will be important to note "usual occupation when working."

---

[9]The SOC has a hierarchical coding structure with 800-plus categories that allows for coding and aggregation at different levels of granularity (BLS, 2010a).

In summary, information on an individual's occupation is often collected and used as a proxy for work-related exposures or potential hazards. The SOC system offers a well-accepted means to standardize these data, and the autocoding applications increase the potential for structuring and using this information for public health surveillance purposes.

BOX 5
Example of the Use of Occupational Data Elements in the EHR:
Work-Related Asthma

Approximately 8 percent of adults in the United States have asthma (Moorman et al., 2011), and nearly 20 percent of new-onset cases in the adult population are estimated to be caused by occupational exposures (Toren and Blanc, 2009). Among adults with asthma, it is estimated that more than 20 percent have symptoms that are exacerbated by conditions at work (Henneberger et al., 2006, 2011). The link between asthma and occupational exposures often goes unrecognized by both clinicians and patients. Failure to identify work-related asthma and reduce exposures to asthma-causing agents results in poorer prognosis (Tarlo et al., 2008). Healthy People 2020 has set as a developmental objective that baseline and tracking data should be collected on whether adults have talked about possible work-relatedness of their asthma with their health care professionals (Healthy People 2020, 2010).

If a patient with wheezing (e.g., a janitor exposed to cleaning products) was seen in a setting where occupational information was collected in the EHR, care could be improved in a variety of ways. Each data element provides insights and opportunities for improving the health care visit but not all are relevant to each visit.

By knowing the industry in which the patient works—for example, if the patient was a school janitor, a janitor in a hospital, or a janitor in some other setting—the clinician would be better able to determine the type and nature of the exposure.

Exposure

If there is a suspected exposure, the clinician could potentially link through the EHR to a website to learn more about frequent exposures in this occupation and industry and determine whether the patient should be evaluated by an occupational health specialist or pulmonologist.

Work-Relatedness

If work-relatedness is suspected, the clinician could access clinical decision-support tools with appropriate treatment guidelines. If the asthma is determined to be caused or exacerbated by work, the clinician could access public health reporting forms (since work-related asthma is a reportable disease in a number of states) that would automatically transmit the case to public health authorities. For return to work, the clinician could recommend that the employer substitute safer cleaning products, provide the worker with appropriate personal protective equipment, or adapt the employee's work practices.

BOX 5 Continued

Employer

If needed, the clinician could write a letter or call the employer to recommend appropriate return-to-work guidelines. Health systems could also choose to look at their internal populations and run de-identified reports on occupation, employer, and work-relatedness in order to guide community outreach and education efforts targeting their patient populations or local employers.

Industry

"Industry" refers to the type of employer or business establishment—for example, auto repair, retail sales, education, health care, or airplane manufacturing. Like occupation, information on the type of industry in which a person works can signal a potential hazardous exposure, especially when coupled with information on specific occupation and employer. Together these pieces of data can improve specificity about the unique potential hazards in the work environment. For example, a janitor in an office building will likely be exposed to different hazards than would a janitor in a manufacturing plant.

Current environment In a number of national health and economics surveys,[10] information on industry is derived from the employer's name. Like "usual occupation," "usual industry" is collected on the standard certificate of death (NCHS, 2003) and is required to be collected when available by all state cancer registries (NAACCR, 2011).

Industry is not generally a data element available in EHRs other than in occupational medicine services. Federal data systems, such as the Census Bureau (2011), rely on the North American Industry Classification System (NAICS), which assigns industry classifications at the establishment level. The type of industry can be derived from the employer's name or from public or private data sources that list NAICS codes. State workforce agencies collect and code information on the employer's industry for all establishments covered by unemployment insurance programs, but it is not clear how or if this information could be made

---

[10]For example, the American Community Survey, the Current Employment Statistics Survey, the Current Population Survey, the Quarterly Census of Employment and Wages, and the Survey of Occupational Injuries and Illnesses.

available for use in EHRs. Other sources of this information, by employer but not employee, are available through sources such as the Dun and Bradstreet (2010) and the National Establishment Time-Series (Walls and Associates, 2011) databases. Coding for industry could be done through the NIOSH autocoder that is under development, if a description of the employer's economic activity, products, or services is available.

Technical considerations   For industry information collected in EHRs to be useful for clinical care, public health surveillance, and research, the same considerations related to collecting and analyzing data on occupation are relevant. A major difference is that, for many workers,[11] information on their designated industry is already available in state workforce agencies' unemployment insurance databases. However, electronic linkage would require matching either on employer name, which can have variations, or a unique employer identifier, such as the Employer Identification Number (EIN). This number is not currently in EHRs, nor is it consistently assigned across business operations. Employees' Social Security numbers (SSNs) could enable a straightforward match if they were available in the EHR; however, there are important privacy concerns regarding SSNs, and current regulations discourage their use.

When coupled with information on a person's occupation, knowing the industry in which he or she works can provide additional insights into potential work exposures or hazards. Further, this data element can be coded for public health surveillance purposes through the NAICS system.

Work-Relatedness

The data element "work-relatedness" denotes the assessment of a link between work and health status. This term is different from other key occupational information in that it is not a separate data element within the EHR. Rather, work-relatedness is a modifier of other data elements, such as symptoms, diagnosis, or exposure, to allow the clinician to denote the relationship between a health event and work risks or exposures. Documentation of work-relatedness in the EHR may facilitate patient management, individual patient access to workers' compensation benefits and other resources, public health reporting of notifiable conditions, and use of data for surveillance of work-related injuries and illnesses.

---

[11]Excluding, for example, self-employed and migrant workers.

Current environment Typically work-relatedness is not known to be documented systematically unless the patient is treated in an occupational health setting or has a clinical encounter in which workers' compensation has been designated as the payer. Work-relatedness may be documented in many sections of the EHR in various formats. Direct or indirect assertions of work-related events may appear as the chief complaint or in the history of present illness, past medical history, social history, problem list, assessment, or treatment plan. The variation in the location and format of this information limits the potential for querying or aggregating work-related events in an EHR. For example, in the Cambridge Health Alliance EHR, suspected work-relatedness can be noted in the problem list (Personal communication, Laura Brightman, Cambridge Health Alliance, July 19, 2011).

Many physicians receive little training in occupational medicine, may not be aware of the effects that specific work exposures can have on health, and may find it challenging to determine whether specific illnesses or disorders are work related. Further, there may be little motivation to document work-relatedness, due to the low reimbursement rates and complex reporting requirements of state workers' compensation programs. Patients likewise may not want work-relatedness to be documented because they do not want to use the workers' compensation system or are otherwise concerned that the association of a condition with work could affect job security. This may particularly impact the reporting decisions of low-wage, immigrant, or contingent workers (Azaroff et al., 2002).

Technical considerations Work-related acute injuries are those that occur during the course of work. The health care professional typically relies on input from the patient or from another party in assessing work-relatedness. Work-related illnesses are those that are either caused or exacerbated by work (WHO Expert Committee, 1985). The patient may judge an illness to be work related; however, a health care professional's assessment is generally necessary to obtain workers' compensation benefits or to confirm reportable work-related conditions.

Although a few diseases, such as silicosis, may be assumed to be related to work, usually work-relatedness must be applied to a specific diagnosis or symptom code. The common coding systems used for billing offer limited support for coding work-relatedness. In the International Classification of Diseases-Ninth Revision (ICD-9) and ICD-9-Clinical Modification (CM), there is a "location of injury" code that is not synonymous with work-relatedness. ICD-10 has added a digit that can be used to code for activity at time of injury, and work activity is one of the options. Furthermore, there are ICD-10 codes that denote work-relatedness for specific exposures and injuries, but none exists for more general or chronic diseases (e.g., diabetes, asthma). ICD-10 is not yet in widespread use in the United States. Designation of workers' compensation as payer in the administrative record also indicates work-relatedness, but fails to capture a substantial proportion of work-related conditions, particularly diseases. Further efforts are needed to explore the best person, place, and time to document work-relatedness in the EHR.

Having a data element or attribute to denote work-relatedness could prompt health care professionals to think about the potential for a connection between work and the health condition. Although more education for clinicians and patients is needed regarding these potential connections, this prompt in the EHR could be one of the starting points for early recognition of an association as well as for further education efforts.

Employer Information

To adequately capture employer information, current employer name and worksite address are necessary. Having both name and address reduces ambiguity about the specific employer and the work environment of the employee and can enable a feedback loop if problems are identified.

Current environment   Information about the patient's employer may be captured in the administrative portion of EHRs for billing and claims purposes. If this information exists in clinical records, it is often in narrative text, as part of the social history. Employer information gathered for administrative purposes may reflect the parent's or spouse's employer and source of health insurance, which can create challenges for health surveillance efforts. High-level employer codes may provide information about the "parent company" for which a person works, but provide little insight about the conditions and exposures in the employee's actual worksite.

In 2009, almost 60 percent of non-elderly individuals in the United States were covered by an employment-based health benefits plan, either through their own employment or as family members of an insured person (Fronstin, 2010). Providing this benefit is costly for U.S. businesses, which has sparked interest in the "development of best approaches to motivate employee/family engagement in improving health and well-being, with measurable results" (National Business Group on Health, 2011). In some EHR systems, such as Dartmouth-Hitchcock's (2011), knowing who the employer is allows clinicians to refer employees to appropriate wellness programs at their own worksite.

Health insurance cards are a potential source of occupational information including employee's occupation, industry, and employer name. Developing ways to integrate this information into the EHR could be explored, as could occupational information available for Medicaid and Medicare beneficiaries.

Technical considerations As noted above, a two-way interface with administrative data elements populating clinical records and vice-versa should be possible so that all parts of the EHR contain uniform, up-to-date employer data. However, synchronization of data across the record may be difficult.

It is possible, but may not be practical, to collect and maintain a history of employer names, worksite addresses, company addresses, and dates of employment. As is the case with many EHR data elements, the usefulness of employer data varies by user. "Employer" may be a critical data element for billing, but only "nice-to-have" for a specific clinician, whereas another clinician may need employer information in text format in order to complete return-to-work forms. Similarly, the specificity desired for epidemiologic purposes is likely different from that needed for billing or clinical care.

To be most useful for both health care and public health, employer information should be standardized and coupled with other information, such as job tasks or potential exposures. Public health applications need employer information aggregated by employer, occupation, and industry. Because a business name and street address can be reported in many different formats, including either trade name or legal name and either with or without abbreviation, this data element can be challenging to link with unique identifiers or map to industry codes for routine surveillance. For limited studies, it could be coded manually.

Recording an EIN, Dun and Bradstreet number, or other identification number would help standardize analysis; however, it is not practical to ask a busy clinician to collect these numbers, and patients would rarely have that information. Provider organizations serving large employers may be able to incorporate unique employer identifiers using human resources data sources. It may be possible to geocode the actual worksite, as identified by the employee on a map, rather than impute it from the address.

Exposures

Accurate information about the chemical, physical, or radiation exposures an employee has experienced would be the most specific, and therefore the most useful, occupational information, although it is the most difficult to obtain. In addition, a worker may be impacted by other types of exposures such as psychological stress. Although it was beyond the committee's scope of work to consider the full range of factors that impact a worker's health, further exploration is needed on how best to collect and use this information in the EHR.

Current environment Documenting exposures can be important in cases of illness, but also in the absence of health conditions if ongoing monitoring is required or advised, or if an exposure (e.g., asbestos) interacts with other risk factors, such as smoking.

Outside of occupational medicine services, information about potentially hazardous chemical or physical exposures is not systematically collected in EHRs. This information can be captured in narrative text fields, in the problem list, or elsewhere in clinical notes. A few coded data structures are available, but not widely used. For example, exposure codes created by the Association of Occupational and Environmental Clinics (AOECs) are searchable online at no cost and include a supplemental set of codes for asthmagens (AOEC, 2011). Approximately one-third of AOEC members in nine states and two Canadian provinces currently use and report data with these codes, as do states conducting NIOSH-sponsored surveillance of sentinel occurrences of work-related asthma (Personal communication, Katherine H. Kirkland, AOEC, July 14, 2011). Another potential source for information on job hazards exists in many large companies, where human resources departments sometimes maintain a job exposures database that could be linked to EHRs for their workers.

Finally, several online resources are currently available with information on the health impacts of hazardous work conditions (see Box 6). These resources could potentially be linked to EHRs (perhaps using the existing Health Level 7 International [HL7] "Infobutton" standard for context-aware information retrieval [Del Fiol et al., 2008]).

> **BOX 6**
> **Examples of Online Databases with Information on**
> **Health Effects of Hazardous Exposures**
>
> - Material Safety Data Sheet (MSDS) databases can be searched by product name (e.g., MSDSonline, 2011).
> - The Haz-Map database developed by the National Library of Medicine contains information on exposure, illness, and jobs (National Library of Medicine, 2011) and has the potential to populate fields with data related to job descriptions.
> - The International Labour Office Encyclopedia of Workplace Health and Safety Information is an online database that contains an extensive array of exposure information for chemical and physical hazards (ILO, n.d.).
> - The ICD-10-CM diagnosis codes Z57.0-9 contain some generic occupational exposure codes (ICD-10, n.d.). There are also codes for the toxic effects of specific (e.g., aflatoxin, sulfur dioxide, lead) and nonspecific (e.g., "toxic effect of unspecified gases, fumes, and vapors") exposures. Additionally, ICD-10-CM external cause of injury codes have a "place of occurrence" digit to indicate workplace risk (WHO, 2006).
> - EXTOXNET, specific to pesticides, can be searched by active ingredient names (EXTOXNET, 2011).

Technical considerations The level of detail needed to alert a clinician about a health risk may be relatively coarse, such as "organic solvent" or "noise." However, to be useful epidemiologically, more detail is needed. Occupation paired with industry does not by itself identify a specific exposure, because different employers may use different chemicals or processes for the same task. Physical hazards may be easier to classify based on job title (such as radiation technician), but these, too, will often require specific questioning before a causal association can be established.

Clinicians in general are unfamiliar with the names or contents of many chemical substances to which workers are exposed. Worker-entered data on their own occupational exposures may be quite broad but, given certain health conditions, may be sufficient to prompt further questions. One initial step may be to ask patients if they have been exposed to hazardous toxins where the association with disease has been well documented (e.g., lead, asbestos) or if they are required to use personal protective equipment, which would indicate exposure risks identified by the employer. Furthermore, workers in workplaces covered by OSHA rules have the right to request information about the chemicals to which they have been exposed. OSHA requires employers to provide their employees, on request, with Material Safety Data Sheets on hazardous chemicals (29 CFR 1910.1200(b)(4)(ii)).

Existing information sources on exposures could be linked to EHRs; however, their value for clinical use needs to be assessed because they are not designed for use by a busy clinician. Standards do exist for context-aware information retrieval (e.g., HL7 [2007]), though this functionality requires that information in the EHR be structured and standardized using codes. These same codes can link exposure information to occupations in the work history as well as clinical decision support. In the short term, it may be useful to provide clinicians with links to general resources, such as the Haz-Map website or the poison control center phone number.

Cross-Cutting Challenges and Opportunities

In addition to the unique considerations for each data element, the committee identified several cross-cutting challenges and opportunities related to the inclusion of occupational information in the EHR. Each of these, if addressed, could facilitate the use of occupational information by busy clinicians who otherwise might be resistant to adding additional data elements into the EHR. The following could improve patient care with regards to occupational health conditions:

- using the EHR problem list to store occupational health information,
- examining the impact on clinical workflow on access to occupational information,
- exploring the feasibility of using patient-entered or validated data, and
- developing ways in which the EHR can support the patient's return to work.

Use of the EHR Problem List

The EHR problem list is one module that could be used to document or highlight information on the work-relatedness of diseases and injuries or on significant exposures that need ongoing monitoring. The Stage 1 meaningful use criteria specify that clinicians should maintain an up-to-date list of current and active diagnoses in a problem list (CMS, 2010c).

If diagnoses could be coded to note that the condition is work related, then the problem list could potentially be used for public health surveillance and research on occupational health. Other enhancements to the problem list could benefit individual health, including documenting exposures and risks, keeping track of and following abnormal laboratory findings, and noting the potential for work to affect recovery from a disease or injury.

Current environment To date, clinicians have not consistently maintained problem lists, with respect to either format or content (Fung et al., 2010; Holmes, 2011). Even when using an EHR, physicians may not use its problem list section and may instead create their own list within the text of a note. Problem lists vary with respect to levels of specificity, describing observations (e.g., an abnormal laboratory test result or physical finding, such as elevated blood pressure) as well as diagnoses. Health care professionals may not take the time to consistently update the problem list to reflect current status of treatment or evolution of the problem. In some health systems, the problem list for an individual patient may be shared across specialties or types of clinicians (M.D./R.N.) or through other mechanisms. If integrated across clinicians, it is unclear who will be able to update an entry made by another health care professional.

Problem lists may be coded or text-based. Coded lists may have modifiers (e.g., acute or chronic, history of . . .) that change the meaning of the code. "Work-related" is a potentially useful modifier that is not typically included in most current EHR systems. The use of the problem list field is becoming more common, due to the mandate to meet meaningful use criteria. In addition to increasing use, this requirement may improve the consistency of the data that are collected since codes such as ICD, SNOMED-CT (Systematized Nomenclature of Medicine—Clinical Terms), or their equivalents are commonly used in the problem list. Currently the ICD-9 is the most commonly used disease/condition coding system, but others also are used, especially by medical subspecialists who have more specific lexicons (e.g., RadLex) (RSNA, 2011). However, standard formats and coding schemes for problem lists were not prescribed by the proposed Stage 2 meaningful use rules (HHS, 2011).

Technical considerations The problem list serves different purposes for different clinicians. For example, a problem list in an ambulatory setting is quite different from that in an acute care setting. Different specialties often need different levels of detail. This contributes to tensions over who "owns" the problem list or the specific problems on it. Deciding who is responsible for maintaining the problem list requires a cross-clinician coordination mechanism that does not currently exist. Some systems use the problem list to assist in coding visits or episodes of care; others auto-populate the problem list with the coded diagnoses obtained for billing. While the latter has the benefit of adding coded data, it may be imprecise (e.g., abnormal lab value versus abnormal lead level), may duplicate problems (e.g., diabetes, poorly controlled diabetes, diabetic retinopathy, diabetic nephropathy), and may not provide a mechanism to remove or update problems over time.

Abnormal findings are only modestly represented as coded diagnoses in the ICD-9 coding system, or even the soon-to-be-implemented ICD-10. A few laboratory test abnormalities that are associated with known diseases, such as abnormal lead levels, have codes, as do the toxic effects of a few specific exposures—for example, to various metals (e.g., mercury, arsenic), solvents (e.g., benzene, carbon disulfide), and gases (e.g., freon, chlorine). Lack of a code could hinder the entry of pertinent findings as problems that need to be tracked. As mentioned, ICD-10 codes will allow coding of work-relatedness for specific exposures and injuries, but not for more general or chronic diseases such as diabetes or asthma. SNOMED-CT is an option with increasing interest, although the multi-axial nature of the terminology, specific content limitations, and usability to physicians unfamiliar with the system present significant challenges to adoption.

Considerations regarding specificity, reliability, validity, ownership, and currency complicate the potential ways that problem lists can be used and exchanged. The ability to note the work-relatedness of a health condition or exposure is feasible, but standardization of the information model across diverse workflows and care settings will be complicated and should be harmonized with other efforts to upgrade problem list maintenance for the EHR.

Impact on Clinical Workflow

Clinical workflow, including even the sequencing of data entry, determines much of the usefulness of the EHR and the burden of automation. For example, if a coded diagnosis is not entered until the end or even after the patient's appointment, then decision-support logic linked to that coding cannot be deployed during the visit. The possibility of using a tiered approach for the collection of occupational information could be explored, in which tier one would be basic data collected initially and higher tiers would offer more granular data or data that become desirable when seeking better understanding of a disease or condition.

Current environment Some aspects of workflow are common across health care settings. For example, nearly all settings begin with a patient identification and registration process. This is typically performed by a registrar or administrative staff person upon the patient's arrival at the point of care. A large quantity of administrative and billing data is gathered during this step that is also used clinically and for downstream research and surveillance. Occupational data are sometimes gathered, such as employer and occupation. The encounter can begin with an interview or with the patient entering information on paper or via a web portal or PHR as discussed below.

Administrative systems use registration data for decision support focused on business matters, such as collection of overdue bills. These same data can be used to drive clinically significant actions in the EHR. For example, if the patient's chief complaint is cough, a different documentation template may be presented than if the complaint were headache. These sophisticated uses of decision-support logic are dependent on what the computer knows at a given point in the workflow. The EHR can alert a physician to drug allergies or interactions, but only if the record already contains coded data about the patient's allergies or other prescriptions.

To date, clinical decision-support tools have not been widely applied to occupational injury and illness, in part because the key variables discussed above are not reliably captured in the EHR. The effectiveness of collecting these data will, in part, be determined by workflow considerations, including when they are captured and by whom. Alternative ways of accomplishing this should be evaluated, in order to compile a set of "best practices."

Feasibility of Using Patient-Entered or Validated Data

Current environment While most EHR information is recorded by administrative staff and clinicians, strategies are increasingly available for patients to enter new information or validate existing information in the EHR. Patients may populate the EHR through electronic data entry forms, a patient portal directly linked to the EHR, or the exchange of information from a PHR independent of the EHR.

Technical considerations One recently documented use of this strategy by Intermountain Healthcare allows patients to access, enter, and update family health history in a patient portal (Intermountain Healthcare, 2010). Once entered, these data are linked to the patient's EHR and available to clinicians. There is value in developing and evaluating similar strategies for obtaining work history. Because the information can be completed at home, independent of a clinical encounter, people may have more time to add details, and better access to information that will increase the history's accuracy. Implementing a work history module would involve defining a model for storing occupational information, developing and testing ways to share the information between record systems, and defining appropriate workflows for validation and verification as data from different sources are combined. Research has shown that computers can assist in history-taking, including medication compliance (Schackman et al., 2009).

Ways the EHR Can Support Return to Work

The addition of occupational information to the EHR could streamline return-to-work decision making and paperwork, thereby increasing clinical efficiency. Regardless of the cause of an illness or injury, a worker with a temporary or permanent impairment that might be exacerbated by work or that would make work difficult needs to be accommodated by the employer.

Current environment Some EHRs include data that could be used to assess the impact that work has on injured or ill workers and could simplify the administrative transactions between health care professionals and employers. However, these data may be scattered throughout the record and may be in narrative rather than coded formats. Some standardized disability and impairment scales exist, but they are generally specific to medical specialties (e.g., neurology, orthopedics) and are aimed primarily at considering the effect of the condition on activities of daily living rather than its effect on work or work's effect on the condition. Return-to-work forms, which guide employers in accommodating the injured or ill worker, are not currently standardized, nor are they integrated into the EHR. Finally, the details of workers' jobs that would be needed in order to tailor guidance on appropriate job modifications are not commonly captured; linking EHRs to O*NET could provide job demand information (National Center for O*NET Development, 2011).

Technical considerations Some of the most critical technical hurdles in obtaining information for return to work relate to the clinical workflow: Who should capture what data, and how should they be alerted to do so? For clinicians who are not trained in occupational health, collecting sufficiently detailed occupational information to create a relevant return-to-work order, when added to other demands on their time, is a challenge.

Current HIE efforts are focused on communication among clinicians, patients, payers, and registries. Little attention has been given to how HIE standards might facilitate communication with employers. Such exchange would raise security and privacy concerns and require adherence to regulations that protect patients from employment discrimination. The potential economic costs and benefits of using HIE in the context of returning to work warrant research. More standards are needed for the structure and exchange of return-to-work data, electronically or otherwise. Determination of such standards is a prerequisite to any judicious mandate for the design and use of these data in EHRs.

Initial Requirements and Information Modeling

A common information model, such as one based on the HL7 Reference Information Model (HL7, 2011), is "an essential foundation for exchanging data between heterogeneous systems, pooling data across institutions for clinical and outcomes research, sharing medical decision-support logic, and sharing patient care applications" (Huff et al., 1995, p. 116). During this study, the committee could identify no consistent and comprehensive model for capturing and presenting occupational information in the EHR. This is a fundamental informatics challenge that limits the value of existing occupational information and puts a brake on expanded uses. Once strategies are developed to collect, share, and update occupational information in a standardized manner, the information can serve many purposes, as described.

An information model provides the framework for defining data elements and their necessary attributes, the relationships among these elements, and the code systems required to support use cases. In addition, information modeling enables the interpretation of data elements in context. For example, occupation and industry could be used as proxies for exposure risk, which could indicate a potential problem, or they could be used as supplementary information or modifiers for a work-related injury, which is an actual problem.

The committee identified two core needs associated with modeling occupational information. First, an information model needs to be developed that can build an occupational history over time and adequately describe a person's usual and current occupation, employment status (e.g., active, retired, unemployed), the industry involved, the name of the employer and the location of work, and a history of exposures. Over the years, patients often have multiple occupations and work in multiple industries, so clarifying the status of each and denoting concepts such as "usual occupation" may be important. Second, the models currently used to document health problems and diagnoses need to be enhanced so that they include attributes that allow documentation that a particular clinical event is work related. At least some of the current strategies should be evaluated to identify best practices and problems to avoid.

The committee identified coding systems (e.g., SOC, NAICS) that could be adopted immediately to standardize key occupational information in EHRs. Occupational history and work-related attributes currently are included in some EHRs, but the usefulness of this information is limited because it not standardized and appears in various locations in the health record.

CONCLUSIONS

Incorporating occupational information in the EHR could contribute to fully realizing the meaningful use of EHRs. This information could enable improved individual and population health care through better-informed diagnoses, more focused treatment plans, and improved and streamlined return-to-work guidance. Additionally, occupational information in EHRs could make notifiable disease and injury reporting more efficient and allow for improved surveillance of hazards in the work environment, reduce workplace risks, and improve population health. However, for the benefits of inclusion of occupational data in the EHR to be fully realized, the relevant privacy and security issues regarding patient information must be addressed.

Over the past decade, much has been done to improve the technological landscape for EHRs and efforts continue to move closer to fulfilling the potential of this technology. Clinicians are becoming more familiar with the use of EHRs but inherent resistance to change can be a challenge in introducing any new elements into structured medical records. Adding occupational information could meet such resistance. Therefore, as these technological changes are made, the challenges that are focused on raising clinician's awareness of the potential impact of work on health (and worksites as an opportunity for health promotion and disease prevention) also need to be addressed. Health care professional training needs to emphasize the use of occupational information in clinical decision making. Office processes and clinical work flows in health care settings need to be examined. Collection of information on a person's occupation and industry may be feasible in most health care settings, but standard processes should be explored and implemented regarding who collects the data, at what point in the workflow, and in what detail. People who collect and maintain these data will need training. Data on occupation and industry will have to be coded, preferably using existing systems to convert narrative text to coded data. Clinical and administrative systems that can "talk to each other" and efficiently exchange information would allow clinicians to verify or flesh out data entered by administrative staff or patients. Finally, standard forms and processes are needed to enable uniform public health case reporting and surveillance.

As discussed throughout this report, the committee considered in depth the five data elements that are commonly used in occupational health data collection and are considered the most useful for clinical and public health purposes—occupation, industry, work-relatedness, employer, and exposures. Of the five that were explored, three elements were deemed ready for immediate focus—occupation, industry, and work-relatedness—with the other two (employer and exposures) requiring more extensive background work on how best to collect and standardize them for clinical and epidemiologic purposes. Both the occupation and the industry data elements have well-accepted standardized coding classification systems and have been used extensively in public health surveillance efforts. The data element for work-relatedness is an attribute that the health care professional can note and that offers an opportunity to link work with the health condition. The incorporation of each of the three proposed data elements should provide essential occupational information that will enhance meaningful use of EHRs to improve quality of health care and population health.

RECOMMENDATIONS

Given the overall objective of recording, maintaining, protecting, and optimally using occupational information in EHRs, the committee has developed a set of recommendations that include feasibility studies, demonstration projects, and other action steps. These efforts need to be explored in a range of care settings (e.g., specialty practices, ambulatory, acute care), with different employee populations, and in different geographic regions. Where possible, alternative strategies for data collection, as well as the time and cost involved, the impact on clinician efficiency and practice, and the significance for health outcomes should be investigated. These efforts will inform the development of performance measures, decision-support logic, codes, and data structures necessary for NIOSH to make the case for ONC to recommend the inclusion of occupational information in the EHR. Most of these efforts involve collaborations with multiple agencies and organizations.

The committee outlines below a set of recommendations for an initial focus on the three data elements—occupation, industry, and work-relatedness—as well as a set of recommendations on efforts that could begin immediately or in phases to develop clinical decision-support tools, put forth evaluation metrics, and enhance the depth of occupational information available in the EHR. EHRs are inherently dynamic, and there will be numerous opportunities for continued improvements in the foreseeable future. The committee's recommendations are intended to provide an ongoing line of reasoning that will support successively more sophisticated inclusion and use of occupational information in EHRs over a period of years.

Initial Focus on Occupation, Industry, and Work-Relatedness Data Elements

Demonstration projects focused on incorporating occupation, industry, and work-relatedness data elements into the EHR will provide NIOSH with the depth of information that is needed to show feasibility for enhancing patient care and public health across a range of care settings and locations. A robust information model will provide the EHR industry with a target for development that can enhance usability and interoperability over time. By promoting specific, existing coding terminologies now, rather than waiting to develop the "ideal" solution, NIOSH can enable the timely inclusion of occupational data in EHRs as part of the meaningful use criteria and processes. An additional part of that effort to facilitate ONC's acceptance of NIOSH's recommendations will be to develop specific performance measures and meaningful use metrics. Issues regarding privacy and access to health information in the context of work-related health will need further exploration.

Recommendation 1: Conduct Demonstration Projects to Assess the Collection and Incorporation of Information on Occupation, Industry, and Work-Relatedness in the EHR

NIOSH, in conjunction with other relevant organizations and initiatives, such as the Public Health Data Standards Consortium and Integrating the Healthcare Enterprise (IHE) International, should conduct demonstration projects involving EHR vendors and health care provider organizations (diverse in the services they provide, populations they serve, and geographic locations) to assess the collection and incorporation of occupation, industry, and work-relatedness data in the EHR at different points in the workflow (including at registration, with the medical assistant, and with the clinician). Further, to examine the bidirectional exchange of occupational data between administrative databases and clinical components in the EHR, NIOSH in conjunction with IHE should conduct an interoperability-testing event (e.g., Connectathon) to demonstrate this bidirectional exchange of occupational information to establish proof of concept and, as appropriate, examine challenges related to variable sources of data and reconciliation of conflicting data.

Recommendation 2: Define the Requirements and Develop Information Models for Storing and Communicating Occupational Information

NIOSH, in conjunction with appropriate domain and informatics experts, should develop new or enhance existing information models for storing occupational information, beginning with occupation, industry, and work-relatedness data and later focusing on employer and exposure data. The information models should consider the various use cases in which the information could be used and use the recommended coding standards. For example, NIOSH should consider how best to use social history templates to collect a work history and the problem list to document exposures and abnormal findings and diagnoses with optional work-associated attributes for possible, probable, or definite causes; exposures; and impact on work.

Recommendation 3: Adopt SOC and NAICS Coding Standards for Use in the EHR

NIOSH, with assistance from other federal agencies, organizations, and stakeholders (e.g., Bureau of Labor Statistics, Census Bureau, Council of State and Territorial Epidemiologists [CSTE], National Library of Medicine, National Institute of Standards and Technology, National Uniform Billing Committee, HL7), should recommend to the Health IT Standards Committee the adoption of SOC and NAICS to code occupation and industry. Furthermore, NIOSH should develop models for reporting health data from EHRs by occupation and industry at different levels of granularity that are meaningful for clinical and public health use.

Recommendation 4: Assess Feasibility of Autocoding Occupational Information Collected in Clinical Settings

NIOSH should place high priority on completing the feasibility assessment of autocoding the narrative information on occupation and, where available, industry that currently is collected and recorded in certain clinical settings, such as the Dartmouth-Hitchcock health care system, Kaiser Permanente, New York State Occupational Health Clinic Network, Cambridge Health Alliance, and hospitals participating in the National Electronic Injury Surveillance System.

Recommendation 5: Develop Meaningful Use Metrics and Performance Measures

Based on findings from the various demonstration projects and feasibility studies, NIOSH, with the assistance of relevant professional organizations and the Health IT Policy Committee, should develop meaningful use metrics and health care performance measures for including occupational information in the meaningful use criteria, beginning with the incorporation of occupation, industry, and work-relatedness data, and later expanding as deemed appropriate to include other data elements such as exposures and employer.

Recommendation 6: <u>Convene a Workshop to Assess Ethical and Privacy Concerns and Challenges Associated with Including Occupational Information in the EHR</u>
NIOSH should convene a workshop involving representatives of labor unions, insurance organizations, health care professional organizations, workers' compensation-related organizations (e.g., International Association of Industrial Accident Boards and Commissions, National Council on Compensation Insurance), and EHR vendors to

- assess the implications for the patient and clinician of incorporating work-relatedness in the EHR, with respect to workers' compensation; and
- propose guidelines and policies for protecting the patient's non-work-related health information from inadvertent disclosure and to ensure compliance with HIPAA, workers' compensation, and other privacy standards.

Enhance the Value and Use of Occupational Information in the EHR

Much can be done to explore innovative approaches to enhance the value of occupational information and use the full capabilities of the EHR for the benefit of individual workers and public health. Evaluation of various methods of collecting occupational information can identify the best methods of achieving efficiency and privacy, while lowering the cost of data collection and improving accuracy. The development of clinician-friendly tools to support clinical decision making, education, and return to work will contribute to greater awareness of the relationship between work and health, inform treatment and improve patient outcomes, and support safer workplaces. The positive impact of including occupational information in the EHR should expand over time, but ongoing research by NIOSH will help document and promote the most valuable changes while helping to identify and avert unintended consequences.

Recommendation 7: <u>Develop and Test Innovative Methods for the Collection of Occupational Information for Linking to the EHR</u>
NIOSH should initiate efforts in collaboration with large health care provider organizations, health insurance organizations, EHR ven-

dors, and other stakeholders to develop and test methods for collecting occupational data from innovative sources. Specifically, NIOSH should evaluate collection methods that involve

- patient input through mechanisms such as web-based portals and PHRs, and
- other means such as health-related smart cards, health insurance cards, and human resource systems.

Recommendation 8: <u>Develop Clinical Decision-Support Logic, Education Materials, and Return-to-Work Tools</u>
NIOSH, relevant professional organizations, and EHR vendors should begin to develop, test, and iteratively refine and expand

- clinical decision-support tools for common occupational conditions (e.g., work-related asthma);
- tools and programs that could be easily accessed for education of patients and caregivers about occupational illnesses, injuries, and workplace safety;
- training modules for administrative staff to collect occupational information in different care settings; and
- tools to improve and standardize functional job assessment and return-to-work documentation in EHRs, including standards for the transmission of these forms.

Recommendation 9: <u>Develop and Assess Methods for Collecting Standardized Exposure Data</u>
NIOSH should continue to work with occupational and environmental health clinics and other relevant stakeholders to develop and assess methods for collecting standardized exposure data for work-related health conditions. NIOSH should explore the feasibility of

- listing possible or probable exposures in the problem list or elsewhere in the EHR;
- linking occupational information in the EHR to online occupational, toxicological, and hazardous materials databases, such as O*NET, AOEC, and Haz-Map, to enhance diagnosis and treatment of work-related illnesses and injuries; and
- automatically generating codes for exposures based on narrative text entries.

Recommendation 10: Assess the Impact of Incorporating Occupational Information in the EHR on Meaningful Use Goals
NIOSH, in conjunction with relevant stakeholders (e.g., Public Health Data Standards Consortium, CSTE, Association of State and Territorial Health Officials), should

- develop measures and conduct periodic studies to assess the impact of integrating occupational information in EHRs, and
- estimate the economic impact of EHR-facilitated return-to-work practices for both work-related and non-work-related conditions.

REFERENCES

AOEC (Association of Occupational and Environmental Clinics). 2011. *Exposure code lookup.* http://www.aoecdata.org/ExpCodeLookup.aspx (accessed July 12, 2011).

Archer, N., U. Fevrier-Thomas, C. Lokker, K. A. McKibbon, and S. E. Straus. 2011. Personal health records: A scoping review. *Journal of the American Medical Informatics Association* 18(4):515-522.

Azaroff, L. S., C. Levenstein, and D. H. Wegman. 2002. Occupational injury and illness surveillance: Conceptual filters explain underreporting. *American Journal of Public Health* 92(9):1421-1429.

BLS. 2010a. *Standard Occupational Classification.* http://www.bls.gov/soc/ (accessed July 14, 2011).

———. 2010b. *Workplace injuries and illnesses—2009.* http://bls.gov/news.release/pdf/osh.pdf (accessed December 23, 2010).

———. 2011a. *American Time Use Survey summary: 2010 results.* http://www.bls.gov/news.release/atus.nr0.htm (accessed July 27, 2011).

———. 2011b. *National Census of Fatal Occupational Injuries in 2010 (preliminary results).* http://bls.gov/news.release/cfoi.nr0.htm (accessed September 1, 2011).

Boden, L. I., and A. Ozonoff. 2008. Capture-recapture estimates of nonfatal workplace injuries and illnesses. *Annals of Epidemiology* 18(6):500-506.

Boden, L. I., N. Nestoriak, and B. Pierce. 2010. *Using capture-recapture analysis to identify factors associated with differential reporting of workplace injuries and illnesses.* http://www.bls.gov/osmr/pdf/st100300.pdf (accessed May 26, 2011).

California Department of Public Health. 2010. *Infectious diseases case report forms.* http://www.cdph.ca.gov/pubsforms/forms/Pages/CD-Report-Forms.aspx#infectious (accessed September 6, 2011).

Census Bureau. 2011. *North American Industry Classification System.* http://www.census.gov/eos/www/naics/ (accessed July 25, 2011).

Church, T. S., D. M. Thomas, C. Tudor-Locke, P. T. Katzmarzyk, C. P. Earnest, R. Q. Rodarte, C. K. Martin, S. N. Blair, and C. Bouchard. 2011. Trends over 5 decades in U.S. occupation-related physical activity and their associations with obesity. *PLoS One* 6(5):e19657.

Clougherty, J. E., K. Souza, and M. R. Cullen. 2010. Work and its role in shaping the social gradient in health. *Annals of the New York Academy of Sciences* 1186(1):102-124.

CMS (Centers for Medicare and Medicaid Services). 2010a. *CMS finalizes requirements for the Medicare electronic health records (EHRs) incentive program.* https://www.cms.gov/apps/media/press/factsheet.asp?Counter=3792&intNumPerPage=10&checkDate=&checkKey=&srchType=1&numDays=3500&srchOpt=0&srchData=&keywordType=All&chkNewsType=6&intPage=&showAll=&pYear=&year=&desc=&cboOrder=date (accessed August 17, 2011).

———. 2010b. *Electronic health records at a glance.* http://www.cms.gov/apps/media/press/factsheet.asp?Counter=3788&intNumPerPage=10&checkDate=&checkKey=&srchType=1&numDays=3500&srchOpt=0&srchData=&keywordType=All&chkNewsType=6&intPage=&showAll=&pYear=&year=&desc=&cboOrder=date (accessed June 20, 2011).

———. 2010c. *Medicare and Medicaid EHR incentive program: Meaningful use Stage 1 requirements summary.* https://www.cms.gov/EHRIncentivePrograms/Downloads/MU_Stage1_ReqSummary.pdf (accessed June 20, 2011).

———. 2011. *CMS EHR meaningful use overview.* http://www.cms.gov/EHRIncentivePrograms/30_Meaningful_Use.asp (accessed June 20, 2011).

Cocchiarella, L. 2011. *Feasibility of occupational health data in the EHR: A clinician's perspective.* PowerPoint presentation at the IOM Workshop on Occupational Information and Electronic Health Records, Washington, DC, June 2. http://iom.edu/~/media/Files/Activity%20Files/Environment/OccupationalHealthRecords/Panel%203%20Cocchiarella.pdf (accessed July 12, 2011).

Colorado Department of Labor and Employment. 2011. *Medical treatment guidelines: Division of workers' compensation.* http://www.colorado.gov/cs/Satellite/CDLE-WorkComp/CDLE/1248095315991 (accessed July 12, 2011).

Crombez, G., J. W. Vlaeyen, P. H. Heuts, and R. Lysens. 1999. Pain-related fear is more disabling than pain itself: Evidence on the role of pain-related fear in chronic back pain disability. *Pain* 80(1-2):329-339.

Del Fiol, G., P. J. Haug, J. J. Cimino, S. P. Narus, C. Norlin, and J. A. Mitchell. 2008. Effectiveness of topic-specific infobuttons: A randomized controlled trial. *Journal of the American Medical Informatics Association* 15(6):752-759.

Dolin, R. H., L. Alschuler, S. Boyer, C. Beebe, F. M. Behlen, P. V. Biron, and A. Shabo Shvo. 2006. HL7 clinical document architecture, release 2. *Journal of the American Medical Informatics Association* 13(1):30-39.

Doyle, T. J., M. K. Glynn, and S. L. Groseclose. 2002. Completeness of notifiable infectious disease reporting in the United States: An analytical literature review. *American Journal of Epidemiology* 155(9):866-874.

Dun and Bradstreet. 2010. *Company look-up*. https://iupdate.dnb.com/iUpdate/companylookup.htm (accessed July 25, 2011).

EXTOXNET. 2011. *EXtension TOXicology NETwork*. http://extoxnet.orst.edu/ghindex.html (accessed July 12, 2011).

Fan, Z. J., D. K. Bonauto, M. P. Foley, and B. A. Silverstein. 2006. Underreporting of work-related injury or illness to workers' compensation: Individual and industry factors. *Journal of Occupational and Environmental Medicine* 48(9):914-922.

Fronstin, P. 2010. *Sources of health insurance and characteristics of the uninsured: Analysis of the March 2010 Current Population Survey*. http://www.Ebri.org/pdf/briefspdf/EBRI_IB_09-2010_No347_Uninsured1.pdf (accessed July 25, 2011).

Frost and Sullivan. 2010. *Smart cards for healthcare in Europe* http://www.frost.com/prod/servlet/market-insight-top.pag?docid=200942088 (accessed August 15, 2011).

Fung, K. W., C. McDonald, and S. Srinivasan. 2010. The UMLS-CORE project: A study of the problem list terminologies used in large healthcare institutions. *Journal of the American Medical Informatics Association* 17(6):675-680.

GAO (Government Accountability Office). 2009. *Enhancing OSHA's records audit process could improve the accuracy of worker injury and illness data*. GAO-10-10. http://www.gao.gov/new.items/d1010.pdf (accessed August 15, 2011).

Guo, H. R., S. Tanaka, L. L. Cameron, P. J. Seligman, V. J. Behrens, J. Ger, D. K. Wild, and V. Putz-Anderson. 1995. Back pain among workers in the United States: National estimates and workers at high risk. *American Journal of Industrial Medicine* 28(5):591-602.

Haz-Map. 2011. *Benzene, aplastic anemia, and leukemia*. http://www.haz-map.com/benzene.htm (accessed August 1, 2011).

Healthy People 2020. 2010. *Healthy People 2020 summary of objectives: Respiratory diseases*. http://www.healthypeople.gov/2020/topicsobjectives2020/pdfs/RespiratoryDiseases.pdf (accessed July 12, 2011).

Henneberger, P. K., S. J. Derk, S. R. Sama, R. J. Boylstein, C. D. Hoffman, P. A. Preusse, R. A. Rosiello, and D. K. Milton. 2006. The frequency of workplace exacerbation among health maintenance organisation members with asthma. *Occupational and Environmental Medicine* 63(8):551-557.

Henneberger, P. K., C. A. Redlich, D. B. Callahan, P. Harber, C. Lemiere, J. Martin, S. M. Tarlo, O. Vandenplas, and K. Toren. 2011. An Official

American Thoracic Society statement: Work-exacerbated asthma. *American Journal of Respiratory and Critical Care Medicine* 184(3):368-378.
HHS (Department of Health and Human Services). 2010. *ONC-authorized testing and certification bodies*. http://healthit.hhs.gov/portal/server.pt?open=512&mode=2&objID=3120 (accessed June 20, 2011).
———. 2011. *HIT Policy Committee: Meaningful use workgroup request for comments regarding meaningful use stage 2*. http://healthit.hhs.gov/media/faca/MU_RFC%20_2011-01-12_final.pdf (accessed May 12, 2011).
Hilaski, H. J. 1981. *Understanding statistics on occupational illnesses.* http://www.bls.gov/opub/mlr/1981/03/art3full.pdf (accessed August 17, 2011).
HL7 (Health Level 7). 2007. *HL7 standards.* http://www.hl7.org/implement/standards/index.cfm?ref=nav (accessed July 12, 2011).
———. 2011. *HL7 Reference Information Model.* http://www.hl7.org implement/standards/rim.cfm (accessed September 6, 2011).
Holmes, C. 2011. The problem list beyond meaningful use. Part I: The problems with problem lists. *Journal of American Health Information Management Association* 82(2):30-33.
Hsu, M. H., J. C. Yen, W. T. Chiu, S. L. Tsai, C. T. Liu, and Y. C. Li. 2011. Using health smart cards to check drug allergy history: The perspective from Taiwan's experiences. *Journal of Medical Systems* 35(4):555-558.
Huff, S. M., R. A. Rocha, B. E. Bray, H. R. Warner, and P. J. Haug. 1995. An event model of medical information representation. *Journal of the American Medical Informatics Association* 2(2):116-134.
ICD-10 (International Classification of Diseases, Tenth Revision). n.d. *ICD-10-CM diagnosis code Z57.0.* http://www.icd10data.com/ICDI0CM/Codes/Z00-Z99/Z55-Z65/Z57-/Z57.0 (accessed July 12, 2011).
ILO (International Labour Office). n.d. *ILO encyclopedia of workplace health and safety information.* http://www.ilocis.org/en/contilo.html (accessed July 16, 2011).
Intermountain Healthcare. 2010. *A patient-entered family health history program.* http://intermountainhealthcare.org/services/genetics/informatics/Pages/ClinicalDataResearch.aspx (accessed July 25, 2011).
IOM (Institute of Medicine). 1988. *The future of public health.* Washington, DC: National Academy Press.
Kliff, S. 2010. The smart set: Could medical information stored on wallet-sized cards cure the country's health-care woes? *Newsweek*, February 16.
Kreiss, K. 2011. *Finding new associations between work and health.* PowerPoint presentation at the IOM Workshop on Occupational Information and Electronic Health Records, Washington, DC, June 2. http://iom.edu/~/media/Files/Activity%20Files/Environment/OccupationalHealth Records/Panel%202%20Kreiss.pdf (accessed July 25, 2011).

Landrigan, P. J., and D. B. Baker. 1991. The recognition and control of occupational disease. *Journal of the American Medical Association* 266(5):676-680.

Lawrence, R. C., D. T. Felson, C. G. Helmick, L. M. Arnold, H. Choi, R. A. Deyo, S. Gabriel, R. Hirsch, M. C. Hochberg, G. G. Hunder, J. M. Jordan, J. N. Katz, H. M. Kremers, and F. Wolfe. 2008. Estimates of the prevalence of arthritis and other rheumatic conditions in the United States. Part II. *Arthritis and Rheumatism* 58(1):26-35.

Luckhaupt, S. E., G. M. Calvert, and M. H. Sweeney. 2011. Documenting occupational history: The value to patients, payers, and researchers. *Journal of the American Health Information Management Association* 82(7):34-37.

McCauley, L. A. 2005. Immigrant workers in the United States: Recent trends, vulnerable populations, and challenges for occupational health. *American Association of Occupational Health Nurses Journal* 53(7):313-319.

McLellan, R. 2011. *Improving the quality of care for the Dartmouth-Hitchcock workforce:The role of occupational health data in the electronic medical record.* PowerPoint presentation at the IOM Workshop on Occupational Information and Electronic Health Records, Washington, DC, June 2. http://iom.edu/~/media/Files/Activity%20Files/Environment/OccupationalHealth Records/Panel%201%20McLellan.pdf (accessed July 12, 2011).

Moorman, J. E., H. Zahran, B. I. Truman, and M. T. Molla. 2011. Current asthma prevalence: United States, 2006-2008. *Morbidity and Mortality Weekly Report Surveillance Summaries* 60(Suppl.):84-86.

MSDSonline. 2011. *MSDS search.* http://www.msdsonline.com/msds-search/ (accessed September 6, 2011).

NAACCR (North American Association of Central Cancer Registries). 2011. *Standards for cancer registries, volume II: Data standards and data dictionary, sixteenth edition.* http://www.naaccr.org/LinkClick.aspx?fileticket=HCCaP9gRXIk%3D&tabid=133&mid=473 (accessed July 25, 2011).

National Business Group on Health. 2011. *Institute on Innovation in Workforce Well-Being.* http://www.businessgrouphealth.org/about/obesity.cfm (accessed July 25, 2011).

National Center for O*NET Development. 2011. *About O*NET.* http://www.onetcenter.org/overview.html (accessed July 14, 2011).

National Library of Medicine. 2011. *Haz-Map: Occupational exposure to hazardous agents.* http://hazmap.nlm.nih.gov/ (accessed July 12, 2011).

National Survey on Drug Use and Health. 2009. *Cigarette use among adults employed full time, by occupational category.* http://oas.samhsa.gov/2k9/170/170Occupation.htm (accessed July 12, 2011).

NCHS (National Center for Health Statistics). 2003. *U.S. Standard certificate of death.* http://www.cdc.gov/nchs/data/dvs/death11-03final-acc.pdf (accessed September 6, 2011).

New York State Workers' Compensation Board. 2010. *New York Mid and Low Back Injury Medical Treatment Guidelines, first edition.* http://www.wcb.

state.ny.us/content/main/hcpp/MedicalTreatmentGuidelines/MidandLowBack InjuryMTG2010.pdf (accessed July 12, 2011).

NIOSH (National Institute for Occupational Safety and Health). 2004. *Preventing lung disease in workers who use or make flavorings.* NIOSH Publication No. 2004-110. Cincinnati, OH: NIOSH. http://www.cdc.gov/niosh/docs/2004-110/ (accessed July 12, 2011).

———. 2011a. *Industry and occupation coding and support: Industry and occupation coding software.* http://www.ced.gov/niosh/topics/coding/software.html (accessed August 15, 2011).

———. 2011b. *NIOSH industry and occupation computerized coding system.* PowerPoint Presentation to the IOM Committee on Occupational Information and Electronic Health Records, June 21, 2011.

Okechukwu, C. A., N. Krieger, G. Sorensen, Y. Li, and E. M. Barbeau. 2009. MassBuilt: Effectiveness of an apprenticeship site-based smoking cessation intervention for unionized building trades workers. *Cancer Causes Control* 20(6):887-894.

Oleinick, A., and B. Zaidman. 2010. The law and incomplete database information as confounders in epidemiologic research on occupational injuries and illnesses. *American Journal of Industrial Medicine* 53(1):23-36.

ONC (Office of the National Coordinator for Health Information Technology). 2010. *Measuring health IT adoption.* http://healthit.hhs.gov/portal/server.pt/community/healthit_hhs_gov__adoption_and_meaningful_use/1152 (accessed August 17, 2011).

Overhage, J. M., S. Grannis, and C. J. McDonald. 2008. A comparison of the completeness and timeliness of automated electronic laboratory reporting and spontaneous reporting of notifiable conditions. *American Journal of Public Health* 98(2):344-350.

Papanek, P. 2011. *Occupational medicine and the EHR.* PowerPoint presentation at the IOM Workshop on Occupational Information and Electronic Health Records, Washington, DC, June 2. http://iom.edu/~/media/Files/Activity%20Files/Environment/OccupationalHealthRecords/Panel%203%20Papanek.pdf (accessed July 12, 2011).

Pransky, G., T. Snyder, A. Dembe, and J. Himmelstein. 1999. Under-reporting of work-related disorders in the workplace: A case study and review of the literature. *Ergonomics* 42(1):171-182.

Rosenman, K. D., A. Kalush, M. J. Reilly, J. C. Gardiner, M. Reeves, and Z. Luo. 2006. How much work-related injury and illness is missed by the current national surveillance system? *Journal of Occupational and Environmental Medicine* 48(4):357-365.

RSNA (Radiological Society of North America). 2011. *RadLex: A lexicon for uniform indexing and retrieval of radiology information resources.* http://www.rsna.org/radlex/ (accessed July 13, 2011).

Ruser, J. W. 2008. Examining evidence on whether BLS undercounts workplace injuries and illnesses. *Monthly Labor Review* August:20-32.

RWJF (Robert Wood Johnson Foundation). 2008. *Issue brief 4: Work and health. Work matters for health.* http://www.commissiononhealth.org/PDF/0e8ca13d-6fb8-451d-bac8-7d15343aacff/Issue%20Brief%204%20Dec%208 2008%20-%20Work%20and%20Health.pdf (accessed June 6, 2011).

Schackman, B. R., Z. Dastur, D. S. Rubin, J. Berger, E. Camhi, J. Netherland, Q. Ni, and R. Finkelstein. 2009. Feasibility of using audio computer-assisted self-interview (ACASI) screening in routine HIV care. *AIDS Care* 21(8):992-999.

Schulte, P. A. 2005. Characterizing the burden of occupational injury and disease. *Journal of Occupational and Environmental Medicine* 47(6):607-622.

Sengupta, I., V. Reno, and John F. Burton, Jr., with the Study Panel on National Data on Workers' Compensation. 2010. *Workers' compensation: Benefits, coverage, and costs, 2008*. Washington, DC: National Academy of Social Insurance.

Silk, B. J., and R. L. Berkelman. 2005. A review of strategies for enhancing the completeness of notifiable disease reporting. *Journal of Public Health Management and Practice* 11(3):191-200.

Smith, G. S., H. M. Wellman, G. S. Sorock, M. Warner, T. K. Courtney, G. S. Pransky, and L. A. Fingerhut. 2005. Injuries at work in the U.S. adult population: Contributions to the total injury burden. *American Journal of Public Health* 95(7):1213-1219.

Sorensen, G., L. Quintiliani, L. Pereira, M. Yang, and A. Stoddard. 2009. Work experiences and tobacco use: Findings from the Gear Up for Health Study. *Journal of Occupational and Environmental Medicine* 51(1):87-94.

Sorensen, G., A. Stoddard, L. Quintiliani, C. Ebbeling, E. Nagler, M. Yang, L. Pereira, and L. Wallace. 2010. Tobacco use cessation and weight management among motor freight workers: Results of the Gear Up for Health Study. *Cancer Causes Control* 21(12):2113-2122.

Souza, K., L. Davis, and J. Shire. 2010a. Chapter 3: Occupational and environmental health surveillance. In *Occupational and environmental health: Recognizing and preventing disease and injury.* Sixth ed., edited by B. S. Levy, D. H. Wegman, S. L. Baron, and R. K. Sokas. New York: Oxford University Press.

Souza, K., A. L. Steege, and S. L. Baron. 2010b. Surveillance of occupational health disparities: Challenges and opportunities. *American Journal of Industrial Medicine* 53(2):84-94.

Staes, C. J., P. H. Gesteland, M. Allison, S. Mottice, M. Rubin, J. H. Shakib, R. Boulton, A. Wuthrich, M. E. Carter, M. Leecaster, M. H. Samore, and C. L. Byington. 2009. Urgent care providers' knowledge and attitude about public health reporting and pertussis control measures: Implications for informatics. *Journal of Public Health Management and Practice* 15(6):471-478.

Steenland, K., C. Burnett, N. Lalich, E. Ward, and J. Hurrell. 2003. Dying for work: The magnitude of U.S. mortality from selected causes of death asso-

ciated with occupation. *American Journal of Industrial Medicine* 43(5):461-482.
Swotinsky, R. 2009. Workers' comp rates under review. *Employer Solutions (Fallon Clinic)* 5(2). http://www.occhealthfallonclinic.org/archive/Newsletterv5n2.htm (accessed August 15, 2011).
Tacci, J. 2011. *Making meaningful change by integrating occupational information in electronic health records: Improving efficiency in clinical practice.* PowerPoint presentation at the IOM Workshop on Occupational Information and Electronic Health Records, Washington, DC, June 2. http://iom.edu/~/media/Files/Activity%20Files/Environment/OccupationalHealthRecords/Panel%201%20Tacci.pdf (accessed July 25, 2011).
Tarlo, S. M., J. Balmes, R. Balkissoon, J. Beach, W. Beckett, D. Bernstein, P. D. Blanc, S. M. Brooks, C. T. Cowl, F. Daroowalla, P. Harber, C. Lemiere, G. M. Liss, K. A. Pacheco, C. A. Redlich, B. Rowe, and J. Heitzer. 2008. Diagnosis and management of work-related asthma: American College of Chest Physicians Consensus Statement. *Chest* 134(3 Suppl.):1S-41S.
Taylor, J. 2011. *Occupational information and health billing records.* PowerPoint presentation at the IOM Workshop on Occupational Information and Electronic Health Records, Washington, DC, June 2. http://www.iom/~/media/Files/Activity%20Files/Environment/OccupationalHealthRecords/Panel%204%20Taylor.pdf (accessed July 25, 2011).
Thomsen, C., J. McClain, K. Rosenman, and L. Davis. 2007. Indicators for occupational health surveillance. *Morbidity and Mortality Weekly Report: Recommendations and Reports* 56(RR-1):1-7.
Toren, K., and P. D. Blanc. 2009. Asthma caused by occupational exposures is common: A systematic analysis of estimates of the population-attributable fraction. *BMC Pulmonary Medicine* 9:7.
Wagner, G. 2011. Engaging patients and their families in care: Workplace wellness. Presentation at the IOM Workshop on Occupational Information and Electronic Health Records, Washington, DC, June 2.
Walls and Associates. 2011. *NETS database by Walls and Associates.* http://www.youreconomy.org/nets/?region=Walls (accessed July 25, 2011).
Wang, S. J., D. W. Bates, H. C. Chueh, A. S. Karson, S. M. Maviglia, J. A. Greim, J. P. Frost, and G. J. Kuperman. 2003. Automated coded ambulatory problem lists: Evaluation of a vocabulary and a data entry tool. *International Journal of Medical Informatics* 72(1-3):17-28.
Ward, M., P. Brandsema, E. van Straten, and A. Bosman. 2005. Electronic reporting improves timeliness and completeness of infectious disease notification, The Netherlands, 2003. *Euro Surveillance* 10(1):27-30.
Washington State Department of Labor and Industries. 2011. *Medical treatment guidelines.* http://www.lni.wa.gov/ClaimsIns/Providers/TreatingPatients/TreatGuide/ (accessed July 12, 2011).

WHO (World Health Organization). 2006. *ICD-10: External causes of morbidity and mortality (V01-Y98)*. http://apps.who.int/classifications/apps/icd/icd10online/index.htm?gv01.htm+s20v01 (accessed July 12, 2011).

WHO Expert Committee. 1985. *Identification and control of work-related diseases. WHO technical report series No. 714.* Geneva, Switzerland: World Health Organization.

Zuroweste, E. 2011. *Migrant Clinicians Network*. PowerPoint presentation at the IOM Workshop on Occupational Information and Electronic Health Records, Washington, DC, June 2. http://iom.edu/~/media/Files/Activity%20Files/Environment/OccupationalHealthRecords/Panel%203%20Zuroweste.pdf (accessed August 24, 2011).

A

Workshop Agenda

Thursday, June 2, 2011

Keck Center of the National Academies
500 Fifth Street, NW
Room 100
Washington, DC

8:00-8:45 a.m.	**Opening Session**

Welcome and Introductions
David Wegman, Chair, Institute of Medicine (IOM) Committee on Occupational Information and Electronic Health Records

Opening Remarks
John Howard, National Institute for Occupational Safety and Health

Discussion

8:45-10:30   **Panel 1: Making Meaningful Change by Integrating Occupational Information in Electronic Health Records**

Facilitators: Laura Obbard and Curtis Cole

Panel Framing Questions:
- *How does capturing occupational data improve care in your area (e.g., by*

improving clinical efficiency and quality, reducing health disparities, engaging patients and families)?
- *With regard to occupational data, what level of specificity is required to effectively inform clinical decision making?*
- *What current evidence or cost savings data are you familiar with that occupational data can impact patient care in each area? How could incorporating this information in an electronic health record (EHR) enhance care?*

8:45-8:50	**Speaker Introductions**
8:50-9:05	**Improving Quality in Clinical Practice** *Robert McLellan*, Dartmouth-Hitchcock Medical Center
9:05-9:20	**Improving Efficiency in Clinical Practice** *James Tacci*, Xerox
9:20-9:35	**Reducing Health Disparities** *Sherry Baron*, National Institute for Occupational Safety and Health (NIOSH)
9:35-9:50	**Engaging Patients and Their Families in Care—Workplace Wellness** *Gregory Wagner*, Mine Safety and Health Administration
9:50-10:30	**Discussion**
10:30-10:45	**Break**
10:45 a.m.-12:15 p.m.	**Panel 2: Opportunities for Public Health Use** **Facilitator:** Robert Harrison Panel Framing Questions: • *What are the challenges of collecting occupational information in electronic*

health records that will be useful for enhancing public health efforts?
- What issues need to be considered so that occupational data in electronic health records will be usable and useful for public health purposes?
- What are your recommendations on next steps?

10:45-10:50	**Speaker Introductions**
10:50-11:05	**Lessons Learned from Using Primary Care Data for Public Health Purposes** *Christie Eheman*, Centers for Disease Control and Prevention (CDC) *Wendy Blumenthal*, CDC
11:05-11:20	**Finding New Associations Between Work and Health** *Kathleen Kreiss*, NIOSH
11:20 a.m.-12:15 p.m.	**Discussion**
12:15-1:00	**Lunch**

1:00-2:45	**Panel 3: Opportunities for Clinical Use**
	
	Facilitators: Sundaresan Jayaraman and Letitia Davis
	
	Panel Framing Questions:
	- *Is occupational information being collected in the EHR in your system?*
	  - *If so, how have these data been used or what is the plan for using this information? What types of occupational information were collected and at what level of specificity?*
	  - *If not, has the collection of occupational information been considered? What could this information bring to your practice? How do you see this*

information being most easily collected and most productively used?
- *What are the challenges of collecting useful occupational information?*
- *What occupational information should be collected so that clinical decision support could be added to the EHR?*

1:00-1:05	**Speaker Introductions**
1:05-1:20	**Occupational Health Clinic Perspective** *Linda Cocchiarella*, Long Island Occupational and Environmental Health Center
1:20-1:35	**Managing Injury and Disease in the Workplace** *Paul Papanek*, University of California, Los Angeles
1:35-2:05	**Primary Care Perspectives** *Edward Zuroweste*, Migrant Clinicians Network *Jack Chapman*, Gainesville Eye Associates (via phone)
2:05-2:45	**Discussion**
2:45-3:00	**Break**
3:00-5:00	**Panel 4: Feasibility—Implementation Issues**

Facilitators: Catherine Staes, Robert Greenes, and George Stamas

Panel Framing Questions:
- *What are the best strategies to ensure that the occupational data being collected are standardized and useful? What level of specificity is required to ensure meaningful use?*
- *What are the challenges and barriers associated with current occupation classification systems? Does the current*

classification system cover all of the occupational information that should be included in electronic health records?
- *What factors are important in determining if and how clinical decision-support tools will be developed and incorporated?*

3:00-3:05	**Speaker Introductions**
3:05-3:20	**Standardization of Terms and Interoperability** *Chris Chute*, Mayo Clinic
3:20-3:35	**Occupational Information and Health Billing Records** *Jennifer Taylor*, Drexel University
3:35-3:50	**Occupation Coding** *Melissa Chiu*, U.S. Census Bureau
3:50-4:05	**Implementation Perspective** *Toby Samo*, AllScripts
4:05-4:20	**Health System Perspective** *Roman Kownacki*, Kaiser Permanente
4:20-5:00	**Discussion**
5:00-5:15	**Concluding Remarks** *David Wegman*
5:15	**Adjourn Workshop**

B

Workshop Participants

Carolyn Bloch
Federal Telemedicine News

Katherine Cox
American Foundation of State, County, and Municipal Employees

Kathleen Fagan
Occupational Safety and Health Administration (OSHA)

Margaret Filios
National Institute for Occupational Safety and Health (NIOSH)

Genny Barkocy Gallagher
NIOSH

Liz Garza
NIOSH

Michael Glass
GlassEye Consulting

Claudia Hix
Day Kimball Hospital

Larry Jackson
NIOSH

Lore Jackson Lee
NIOSH

Phil Morris
Federal Health Initiatives

Stephen Newell
Mercer

Minda Nieblas
OSHA

Patrick O'Connor
American College of Occupational and Environmental Medicine (ACOEM)

Cindy Post
CentriHealth, Inc.

Mary Rubino
Health Affairs

Anita Samuel
Association of State and
 Territorial Health Officials

Teresa Schnorr
NIOSH

Larry Shaughnesy
Contractor to TRICARE

Rosemary Sokas
OSHA

Kerry Souza
NIOSH

Eileen Storey
NIOSH

Marie Sweeney
NIOSH

Andrew Thacher
ACOEM

Umesh Thakkar
U.S. Department of
 Veterans Affairs

David Weissman
NIOSH

Chris Wolfkiel
ACOEM

Theodore Yee
OSHA

Speakers

Sherry Baron
NIOSH

Wendy Blumenthal
Centers for Disease Control and
 Prevention (CDC)

Jack Chapman
Gainesville Eye Associates (via
 phone)

Melissa Chiu
U.S. Census Bureau

Chris Chute
Mayo Clinic

Linda Cocchiarella
Long Island Occupational
 and Environmental Health
 Center

Christie Eheman
CDC

John Howard
NIOSH

Roman Kownacki
Kaiser Permanente

Kathleen Kreiss
NIOSH

Robert McLellan
Dartmouth-Hitchcock
 Medical Center

APPENDIX B

Paul Papanek
University of California, Los Angeles

Toby Samo
AllScripts

James Tacci
Xerox

Jennifer Taylor
Drexel University

Gregory Wagner
Mine Safety and Health Administration

Edward Zuroweste
Migrant Clinicians Network

Committee Members

David H. Wegman (*Chair*)
University of Massachusetts, *emeritus*

Laura O. Brightman
Cambridge Health Alliance

Curtis L. Cole
Weill Cornell Physicians

Letitia K. Davis
Massachusetts Department of Public Health

Robert A. Greenes
Arizona State University

Lawrence Hanrahan
Wisconsin Division of Public Health

Robert Harrison
University of California, San Francisco

Sundaresan Jayaraman
Georgia Institute of Technology

Matthew Keifer
Marshfield Clinic Research Foundation

Catherine Staes
University of Utah School of Medicine

George Stamas
Bureau of Labor Statistics

Institute of Medicine Staff

Cathy Liverman
Program Director

Andrea Schultz
Program Officer

Lara Andersen
Research Associate

Judy Estep
Program Associate

Andrew Pope
Board on Health Sciences Policy Director

C

Committee Biographies

DAVID H. WEGMAN, M.D., M.Sc., is professor emeritus in the School of Health and Environment at the University of Massachusetts, Lowell. Dr. Wegman was appointed professor and founding chair of the Department of Work Environment in 1987. He served a 5-year term as dean of the School of Health and Environment (2003-2008), after which he returned to the faculty until his retirement at the end of 2009. He continues to serve as adjunct professor at the Harvard School of Public Health. He received his B.A. from Swarthmore College and his M.D. and M.Sc. from Harvard University; he is board-certified in preventive medicine (occupational medicine). Previously he served as director of the Division of Occupational and Environmental Health at the University of California, Los Angeles, School of Public Health and on the faculty at Harvard School of Public Health. Dr. Wegman has focused his research on epidemiologic studies of occupational respiratory disease, musculoskeletal disorders, and cancer and has published more than 200 articles in the scientific literature. He has also written on public health and policy issues concerning hazard and health surveillance, methods of exposure assessment for epidemiologic studies, the development of alternatives to regulation, and the use of participatory methods to study occupational health risks. He has served as chair of the National Research Council-Institute of Medicine (NRC-IOM) Committees on Health and Safety Needs of Older Workers and the Health and Safety Consequences of Child Labor, as well as the Committee to Review the NIOSH (National Institute of Occupational Safety and Health) Research Programs. He has also been a member of the NRC-IOM Panel on Musculoskeletal Disorders and Work, the IOM Committees to Review the Health Consequences of Service During the Persian Gulf War and to Review Gender Differences in Susceptibility to Environmental Factors. He is currently chair of the NRC Committee on External Evaluation of NIDRR (National Institute of Disability and Rehabilitation Research) and Its Grantees.

LAURA O. BRIGHTMAN, M.D., is an internist at Cambridge Health Alliance and clinical instructor in medicine at Harvard Medical School. Dr. Brightman works at the Broadway Community Health Center and has been involved in a study to collect and record information about occupation and work-relatedness in its electronic health record system. Dr. Brightman received her M.D. from the University of Pittsburgh School of Medicine.

CURTIS L. COLE, M.D., is the chief information officer at Weill Cornell Medical College, where he is responsible for the core information services that support the research, clinical, education, and administrative functions of the college. Previously, as chief medical information officer he led the implementation of a new electronic medical record system. He is also actively involved in the development of computer systems that support Clinical Research and Terminology Services. Dr. Cole is a graduate of Bowdoin College and received his medical degree from Cornell University Medical College in 1994. He completed his internal medicine residency program at the New York Hospital in 1997. After residency Dr. Cole continued at New York-Presbyterian Hospital-Weill Cornell as a clinical investigator in medical informatics. He also completed a course in leadership development of physicians in academic health centers in 1999 at Harvard University. In 2002, Dr. Cole participated in the Kellogg School of Business, Northwestern University, Executive Development Program. Dr. Cole has several active research projects including participation in the national VIVO consortium. VIVO is a semantic web-based system to help researchers find one another though a national network.

LETITIA K. DAVIS, Sc.D., EdM., is Director of the Occupational Health Surveillance Program in the Massachusetts Department of Public Health where she has worked for over 25 years to develop state-based surveillance systems for work-related illnesses and injuries. She has overseen the formation of a physician reporting system for occupational disease, the Massachusetts Occupational Lead Registry, a comprehensive surveillance system for fatal occupational injuries, the Massachusetts Sharps Injury Surveillance System, and a model surveillance system for work-related injuries to children and adolescents less than 18 years of age. She has conducted numerous surveillance research studies exploring use of existing public health data sources to document work-related injuries and illnesses and is currently engaged in a project incorporating occupational information in the electronic records systems of community health centers to improve documentation occupational health needs of underserved worker populations. She is also responsible for the development of prevention programs to address identified occupational health problems and advises the Department leadership on matters of occupational health policy. Dr. Davis serves as adjunct faculty of the Department of Work Environment at the University of Massachusetts at Lowell and as an instructor at the Harvard School of Public Health. She is also a lead consultant in occupational health to the Council of State and Territorial Epidemiologists and has played a leadership role nationally in the effort integrate occupational health into public health practice at the state level. She is a past member of the Board of Scientific Counselors of the National Institute for Occupational Safety and Health and of the National Advisory Committee on Occupational Safety and Health and currently serves on the national Advisory Committee on Construction Safety and Health. Dr. Davis received her doctorate in Occupational Health from the Harvard School of Public Health in 1983.

ROBERT A. GREENES, M.D., is chair of the Department of Biomedical Informatics at Arizona State University (ASU). Before coming to ASU, Dr. Greenes spent many years at Harvard, in the field of biomedical informatics, first at Massachusetts General Hospital, then at Brigham and Women's Hospital, where he established the Decision Systems Group in 1980 and developed it into a leading biomedical informatics research and development program. Dr. Greenes was professor of radiology and of health sciences and technology at Harvard Medical School and professor of health policy and management at Harvard School of Public Health. For more than 20 years, he has directed the Biomedical Informatics Research Training Program, with support from the National Library of Medicine and other sources, with co-directors now representing 10 hospital and university-based informatics groups throughout the Boston area. Dr. Greenes is a practicing radiologist. His research has been in the areas of clinical decision support, in terms of models and approaches to decision making, the knowledge representation to support it, and its clinical application and validation. He has also been active in the promulgation of standards and fostering of group collaborative work, particularly in knowledge management. A related research interest is human-computer interaction, particularly with respect to the use of clinical information systems by providers and patients, the improved capture of clinical data, and the incorporation of individualized, context-specific decision support. Dr. Greenes is a member of the IOM and served on the IOM Committee on New Approaches to Early Detection of Breast Cancer.

LAWRENCE HANRAHAN, Ph.D., M.S., is chief epidemiologist and director of Public Health Informatics at the Wisconsin Division of Public Health. In this role, he oversees the development of epidemiologic information systems by providing scientific leadership to integrate—on a secure web platform—statewide public health informatics, epidemiology, and surveillance programs. He has more than 31 years' experience in directing and developing statewide electronic public health surveillance systems and epidemiologic investigations. His research interests include occupational and environmental health surveillance, epidemiologic investigation, multivariate analysis, data mining, and public health informatics. He recently led a Robert Wood Johnson Foundation-funded project to determine the information systems requirements for chronic disease surveillance, including the use of clinical electronic medical record data. He participates in several public health informatics forums, including the Association of State and Territorial Health Officials Public Health Informatics Policy Committee, the Public Health Data Standards Consortium, and the CSTE Informatics Team; he served on the Centers for Disease Control and Prevention's (CDC's) Informatics Board of Scientific Counselors. He is an adjunct professor in the Department of Population Health Sciences, University of Wisconsin School of Medicine and Public Health. He has been with the Division of Public Health since 1979 and holds both a master of science and a doctorate degree in epidemiology from the University of Wisconsin, Madison.

ROBERT HARRISON, M.D., M.P.H., is chief of the Occupational Health Surveillance Program of the California Department of Public Health and clinical professor of medicine at the University of California, San Francisco (UCSF). He lectures at the University of California, Berkeley, School of Public Health on environmental diseases and teaches nursing and occupational medicine residents at UCSF. He founded the UCSF Occupational Health Services and was the medical director of the employee health services for many years. Dr. Harrison is the principal investigator of the NIOSH-CDC cooperative agreement for state-based occupational safety and health surveillance in California. He has conducted numerous workplace investigations of work-related asthma, tuberculosis, pesticide illness, carpal tunnel syndrome, workplace fatalities, and blood-borne pathogen exposures. Dr. Harrison received his M.D. degree from the Albert Einstein College of Medicine and his M.P.H. degree from the University of California, Berkeley. He is board-certified in both internal medicine and occupational medicine.

SUNDARESAN JAYARAMAN, Ph.D., is the Kolon Professor in the School of Materials Science and Engineering and in the College of Management at the Georgia Institute of Technology in Atlanta. He and his research students have made significant contributions in enterprise architecture and modeling methodologies for information systems; engineering design of intelligent textile structures and processes; and design and development of knowledge-based systems for textiles and apparel. His group's research has resulted in the realization of the world's first Wearable Motherboard or Smart Shirt. He is currently engaged in studying the role of management and technology innovation in health care. He was involved in the design and development of TK!Solver, the first equation-solving program from Software Arts, Inc., Cambridge, Massachusetts. Dr. Jayaraman worked as a product manager at Software Arts, Inc., and at Lotus Development Corporation in Cambridge before joining Georgia Tech. Professor Jayaraman is a recipient of the 1989 Presidential Young Investigator Award from the National Science Foundation for his research in the area of computer-aided manufacturing and enterprise architecture. He has served on several IOM and NRC committees, including the Committee on Personal Protective Equipment for Healthcare Workers During an Influenza Pandemic, the Standing Committee on Personal Protective Equipment for Workplace Safety and Health, and the Board on Manufacturing and Engineering Design. He received his B.Tech. and M.Tech. degrees from the University of Madras, India, and his Ph.D. from North Carolina State University.

MATTHEW KEIFER, M.D., M.P.H., is senior research scientist and the Dean Emanuel Endowed Chair in Agricultural Medicine at the Marshfield Research Foundation in Wisconsin. He is a senior scientist with the National Farm Medicine Center and remains an affiliate professor of environmental and occupational health sciences at the University of Washington. Dr. Keifer was formerly co-director of the Pacific Northwest Agricultural Safety and Health Center, where he directed numerous community-based research projects that largely focused on farmworker health and pesticides. Dr. Keifer is board-certified in internal medicine and occupational and environmental medicine. His clinical practice is conducted at the Occupational Medicine Clinic at the Marshfield Clinic. Prior to joining the faculty at Washington, he was the regional pesticide epidemiologist in Leon, Nicaragua, from 1989 to 1991, supported by CARE International. Dr. Keifer received his medical training at the University of Illinois and his M.P.H. from the University of Washington.

CATHERINE STAES, B.S.N., M.P.H., Ph.D., is assistant professor of biomedical informatics in the Department of Biomedical Informatics at the University of Utah School of Medicine. Dr. Staes received her Ph.D. in medical informatics from the University of Utah in 2006, a master's in public health from Johns Hopkins University in 1987, and a bachelor of science in nursing from Georgetown University in 1981. Dr. Staes was an Epidemic Intelligence Service officer with the Centers for Disease Control and Prevention (1990-1992), worked as a public health epidemiologist for 15 years, and has numerous publications concerning epidemiology and biomedical informatics. Currently, Dr. Staes' research and teaching focus on the domain of public health informatics and the development of decision-support tools and applications to support surveillance and public health goals. Dr. Staes has broad experience as a public health epidemiologist and has performed research in environmental health (particularly prevention of lead poisoning), communicable disease control, and injury control

GEORGE STAMAS, M.Sc., is chief of the Division of Occupational Employment Statistics at the Bureau of Labor Statistics (BLS) in the U.S. Department of Labor. Mr. Stamas is responsible for the BLS Occupational Employment Statistics (OES) program, a large employer survey collecting data on employment and wages by occupation. He also serves on the Standard Occupational Classification (SOC) Policy Committee.